Treating Schizophrenia in the Prodromal Phase

© 2004 Taylor & Francis, an imprint of the Taylor & Francis Group

First published in the United Kingdom in 2004
by Taylor & Francis, an imprint of the Taylor & Francis Group, 11 New Fetter Lane, London EC4P 4EE

Tel.:   +44 (0) 20 7583 9855
Fax.:   +44 (0) 20 7842 2298
E-mail: info@dunitz.co.uk
Website: http://www.dunitz.co.uk

Although every effort has been made to ensure that all owners of copyright material have been acknowledged in this publication, we would be glad to acknowledge in subsequent reprints or editions any omissions brought to our attention.

Although every effort has been made to ensure that drug doses and other information are presented accurately in this publication, the ultimate responsibility rests with the prescribing physician. Neither the publishers nor the authors can be held responsible for errors or for any consequences arising from the use of information contained herein. For detailed prescribing information or instructions on the use of any product or procedure discussed herein, please consult the prescribing information or instructional material issued by the manufacturer.

A CIP record for this book is available from the British Library.

Library of Congress Cataloging-in-Publication Data

Data available on application

ISBN 1 84184 443 8 (hbk)
ISBN 1 84184 327 X (pbk)

Distributed in North and South America by
Taylor & Francis
2000 NW Corporate Blvd
Boca Raton, FL 33431, USA

Within Continental USA
Tel.: 800 272 7737; Fax.: 800 374 3401
Outside Continental USA
Tel.: 561 994 0555; Fax.: 561 361 6018
E-mail: orders@crcpress.com

Distributed in the rest of the world by
Thomson Publishing Services
Cheriton House
North Way
Andover, Hampshire SP10 5BE, UK
Tel.: +44 (0)1264 332424
E-mail: salesorder.tandf@thomsonpublishingservices.co.uk

Composition by 𝐓 TekArt

Printed and bound in Great Britain by the Cromwell Press Ltd, Trowbridge, Wilts.

Contents

Acknowledgements

To our families.

Foreword

Psychosis generally, and schizophrenia in particular, is a strange and sometimes awful disorder. For many of us researching into psychotic illnesses, it was the strangeness which first attracted us. The extraordinary symptoms seem to reflect on some central core of human experience. Only when one starts to work with people suffering from schizophrenia in its chronic stages do the devastating effects on sufferers and their families begin to strike home. Traditional mental health settings are largely inhabited by people afflicted by the chronic disabling effects of the disorder. One result of training and working in such settings, as many of us do, is an increasing bias to view the disorder as inherently chronic and disabling.

The Melbourne team have overseen a paradigm shift in mental health. Starting with a re-emphasis of the importance of early detection and intervention in psychotic disorders, the group has assembled an interlocking programme of research and therapy since the late 1980s, which covers a variety of areas related to early psychosis. This book describes the origins, rationale and development of potentially the most exciting and important of these areas. In the 1990s, Alison Yung and Patrick McGorry, with Lisa Phillips, delineated a set of operational criteria to identify people at 'ultra high risk' of developing full psychosis within the next year. These criteria were driven by a 'close-in' strategy which sought to combine a range of risk factors in order to identify individuals at the highest risk of psychosis. Crucially, the criteria developed are plausibly open to intervention, pointing to the holy grail of any disorder: its primary prevention.

This book tells the story of how this new focus emerged, reviewing from a first hand perspective the historical context, conceptual issues, research evidence, ethics and the practicalities of setting-up and running a treatment service. The Personal Assessment and Crisis Evaluation (PACE) clinic opened its doors to people with at risk mental states in 1994. The first such service in the UK was set up nearly 10 years later and similar services and research programmes have now started around the world. The Melbourne approach is a benchmark in that it combines an innovative service with active multidisciplinary research, both into the treatment of, and the nature and pathogenesis of, these ultra high risk (sometimes called 'prodromal') states. It is no overstatement to say that research in this area potentially holds the keys to unlocking much of the mystery of psychosis. The very existence of these sub-clinical mental states forces a discussion on the nature of psychosis itself. Is there really a step change in symptom severity which defines categorically a psychosis? Or are we after all dealing with a continuously distributed range of phenomenology which incurs distress or impaired functioning once an individually-set threshold of severity is passed?

There is another important focus here which must not be overlooked: the focus on young people. John Keats, at the start of his poem Endymion (the one which states 'A thing of beauty is a joy forever') says this:

'The imagination of a boy is healthy and the mature imagination of a man is healthy; but there is a space of life in between, in which the soul is in a ferment, the character undecided, the way of life uncertain ....'

The importance of this focus, as emphasised in this book, cannot be underestimated.

Professor Shôn Lewis
Professor of Psychiatry, School of Psychiatry and Behavioural Sciences, University of Manchester, UK

Introduction—an overview

A journey of a thousand miles begins with a single step.
Chinese proverb

1

Preventive strategies in mental health have been a long time coming. Schizophrenia has seemed like the hardest target—particularly, as up until recently, there have been few effective treatments available and ongoing disability was seen as inevitable. However, an earlier generation of clinicians and researchers speculated on the possibility of intervening prior to the onset of acute psychosis—during the *prodrome*. It was thought that providing very early intervention— before the condition became intractable—could minimize the disability and upheaval that an individual and his or her family might have otherwise suffered (Meares, 1959; Sullivan, 1927, reprinted 1994). More than fifty years later, these ideas are becoming translated into real-world practice. What seemed like a giant leap forward to those earlier psychiatrists has become a series of achievable steps with some already behind us.

The possibility of providing treatment prior to the onset of the acute phase of psychotic disorders has arisen from recent growing international interest in early intervention in these disorders (Edwards and McGorry, 2002; Malla and Norman, 2002). Such interest has resulted in the development of strategies for the intensive treatment of the first psychotic episode (Birchwood et al 1998; Edwards et al 1994; Edwards and McGorry, 1998; Falloon et al 1998; McGlashan, 1998; McGorry, 1998; McGorry and Jackson, 1999; Power et al 1998) and improvements in its detection, thus minimizing the delay between onset of psychosis and treatment (Harrigan et al 2003; Larsen and Opjordsmoen, 1996; Lieberman and Fenton, 2000; McGorry, 2000).

This book describes principles and progress in the detection, engagement and treatment of young people with incipient psychosis, as well as summarizing the research findings to date.

Chapter 2 details the significance of the initial prodromal phase for prevention and early intervention in psychosis. Chapter 3 describes the conceptual and background issues necessary before a programme of pre-psychotic intervention is embarked upon.

Chapters 4 and 5 address the more practical issues of setting up a service for potentially 'prodromal' individuals and the particular clinical needs of this patient population. Chapters 6 and 7 describe the research background and study results to date in our programme of clinical research in the pre-psychosis field. Finally, Chapter 8 discusses possible future directions.

Terminology

It is important to state at the outset that frank or full-blown psychosis is the target for the predictive and preventive efforts discussed in this book, rather than schizophrenia *per se*. This is because the onset of a positive psychosis syndrome is an important stage in the development of schizophrenia (Heinssen et al 2001). However, not all first psychotic episodes develop into schizophrenia. Schizophrenia is a subset or subsidiary target. In fact, the broader first episode psychosis target is a more proximal and therapeutically salient one than schizophrenia, which can be considered a subtype to which some patients progress following the first episode of psychosis (McGorry et al 2003). Hence, we acknowledge that we are likely to be predicting and monitoring the onset of a range of disorders. But then, schizophrenia itself represents a heterogeneous range of illnesses, with marked variability in symptoms and outcome. The best we can do is to assess our

target syndrome (full-blown psychosis) and evaluate it concurrently with the present diagnostic systems for more distal disorders, such as schizophrenia.

The young people who have come to see us for assistance and who have been generous in their time and have allowed us to learn from them are referred to throughout the book as *patients*. This term reflects the fact that we work within a public health setting where people with mental health difficulties are commonly referred to as patients. We hope that this does not cause offence. We have provided a number of case studies to illustrate our work. Pseudonyms have been used throughout the book.

The origins of this book and acknowledgements

In writing this book we have drawn on our collective experience from working in the Personal Assessment and Crisis Evaluation (PACE) Clinic, a combined clinical and research centre specifically established to monitor and treat young people suspected of being at high risk for imminent onset frank psychosis (Yung et al 1996). Financial support for the Clinic has come from a number of sources, to whom we are extremely grateful: National Health and Medical Research Council, Department of Health and Human Services (Victoria), the Federal Department of Health and Aging (Australia), Victorian Health Promotion Foundation, Stanley Foundation, Australian Rotary Health Research Fund, Janssen-Cilag Pharmaceuticals, Victor Hurley Research Foundation, and the National Alliance for Research on Schizophrenia and Depression.

We would like to thank our numerous colleagues who have contributed to our research and clinical endeavours over the last decade, in particular, Dr Gregor Berger, who made a major contribution to Chapter 7. Finally, of course, we thank our patients, from whom we have learnt so much.

References

Birchwood M, Todd P, Jackson C (1998) Early intervention in psychosis: The critical period hypothesis. *Br J Psychiatry* **172**(suppl 33):53–59.

Edwards J, McGorry PD (1998) Early intervention in psychotic disorders: A critical step in the prevention of psychological morbidity. In Perris CEM, McGorry PD, eds, *Cognitive psychotherapy of psychotic and personality disorders: Handbook of theory and practice.* Chichester, UK: Wiley: 167–195.

Edwards J, McGorry PD (2002) *Implementing early intervention in psychosis: A guide to establishing early psychosis services.* London: Martin Dunitz.

Edwards J, Francey SM, McGorry PD, Jackson HJ (1994) Early psychosis prevention and intervention: Evolution of a comprehensive community-based specialised service. *Behav Change* **11**:223–233.

Falloon IRH, Coverdale JH, Laidlaw TM, et al (1998) Early intervention for schizophrenic disorders: Implementing optimal treatment strategies in routine clinical services. *Br J Psychiatry* **172**(suppl 33):33–38.

Harrigan SM, McGorry PD, Krstev H (2003) Does treatment delay in first-episode psychosis really matter? *Psychol Med* **33**:97–110.

Heinssen R, Perkins DO, Appelbaum PS, Fenton WS (2001) Informed consent in early psychosis research: National Institute of Mental Health Workshop, November 15, 2000. *Schizophr Bull* **27**:571–584.

Larsen TK, Opjordsmoen S. (1996) Early identification and treatment of schizophrenia: conceptual and ethical considerations. *Psychiatry* **59**:371–380.

Lieberman JA, Fenton WS (2000) Delayed detection of psychosis: Causes, consequences, and effect on public health. *Am J Psychiatry* **157**:1727–1730.

Malla AK, Norman RMG (2002) Early intervention in schizophrenia and related disorders: Advantages and pitfalls. *Curr Opin Psychiatry* **15**:17–23.

McGlashan TH (1998) Early detection and intervention of schizophrenia: Rationale and research. *Br J Psychiatry* **172**(suppl 33):3–6.

McGorry PD (1998) 'A stitch in time…' The scope for preventive strategies in early psychosis. *Eur Arch Psychiatry Clin Neurosci* **248**:22–31.

McGorry PD (2000) Evaluating the importance of reducing the duration of untreated psychosis. *Aust NZ J Psychiatry* **34**(suppl):S145–S149.

McGorry PD Jackson HJ, eds (1999) *Recognition and management of early psychosis: A preventive approach.* Cambridge University Press.

McGorry PD, Yung AR, Phillips LJ (2003) The 'close-in' or ultra high risk model: A safe and effective strategy for research and clinical intervention in prepsychotic mental disorder. *Schizophr Bull* **29**: 771–790.

Meares A (1959) The diagnosis of prepsychotic schizophrenia. *Lancet* **I**:55–59.

Power P, Elkins K, Adlard S, et al (1998) Analysis of the initial treatment phase in first-episode psychosis. *Br J Psychiatry* **172**(suppl 33):71–76.

Sullivan HS (1927, reprinted 1994) The onset of schizophrenia. *Am J Psychiatry* **151**:135–139.

Yung AR, McGorry PD, McFarlane CA, et al (1996) Monitoring and care of young people at incipient risk of psychosis. *Schizophr Bull* **22**:283–303.

The significance of the prodrome for prevention and early intervention

2

I feel certain that many incipient cases might be arrested before the efficient contact with reality is completely suspended, and a long stay in institutions made necessary.

Sullivan 1927 (reprinted 1994: 135)

What is needed is not the early diagnosis of schizophrenia but the diagnosis of prepsychotic schizophrenia. We must learn to recognise that state of mind which will develop into schizophrenia unless appropriate measures are taken to prevent deterioration.

Meares (1959: 55)

The prevention or delay of schizophrenia and Alzheimer's Disease are among the most urgent moral, social, economic, public health, and scientific imperatives of our time. Should preventive efforts succeed against these twin (and possibly related) scourges of the young and the old respectively, the fate of humankind would be forever enhanced.

Post (2001: 104)

As these extracts illustrate, the idea of intervening early to prevent the onset of schizophrenia and related disorders is not new. As this chapter will discuss, the pre-psychotic or prodromal phase is a potential target for such preventive treatment.

The prodrome is symptomatic and potentially detectable

The period prior to a clear-cut diagnosis of a psychotic disorder, such as schizophrenia, has traditionally been referred to as the 'premorbid phase'. However, this term has led to some confusion because it actually covers two phases, not one: the true premorbid phase and the prodromal phase or prodrome. The distinction between these two phases is illustrated in Figure 2.1.

The term 'prodrome' is derived from the Greek word *prodromos*, meaning the forerunner of an event (Fava and Kellner 1991). It is a concept commonly used in clinical medicine and refers to the early symptoms and signs that a person experiences before the full-blown syndrome of an illness becomes evident. Thus, the term 'prodrome' has two implications: (1) the person is symptomatic during this phase; and (2) the person will develop a full-blown illness following the prodrome. These two points are both relevant to our thinking about identifying and providing treatment for people suspected of being in the prodromal phase of a first psychotic episode. First, because individuals experiencing a prodrome are symptomatic it means that they may seek help at this stage for their problems and may therefore be detectable. Second, the implication that they will invariably develop the full-blown illness highlights the fact that the prodrome is a retrospective concept. It can only really be recognized after the definitive disorder has begun. These two issues might seem paradoxical, but this is not the case, as the reader will see as this discussion continues.

Various studies comparing controls and individuals who later developed schizophrenia have demonstrated some significant differences

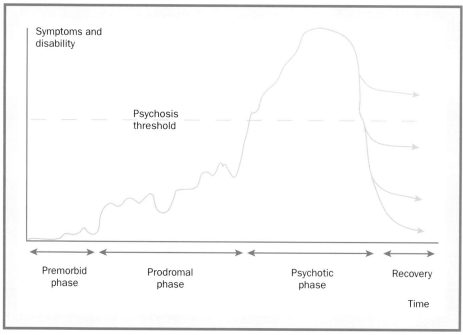

Figure 2.1
Distinctions between the premorbid, prodromal and psychotic phases of a first episode of psychosis.

between the groups during childhood, such as: social adjustment, achievement of milestones of motor development, social anxiety and speech difficulties with the later schizophrenia group performing worse (Done et al 1994; Jones et al 1994). These differences are subtle and highlight the relative quiescence of the illness during childhood. These studies, and the findings of Häfner and colleagues revealed that psychotic illnesses really begin to have clinical and social consequences after puberty, typically during adolescence and early adult life (Häfner et al 1995). This prodromal phase is characterized by non-specific symptoms and growing functional impairment. In fact, a very substantial amount of the disability that develops in schizophrenia accumulates prior to the appearance of the full positive psychotic syndrome (Agerbo et al 2003; Häfner et al 1995; Yung and McGorry 1996). It has even been proposed that the disability, which develops during the prodrome, may create a ceiling for eventual recovery in young people (McGorry et al 2003).

There is now evidence that at some point in transition from prodromal state to full-blown psychotic disorder alterations in brain structure (and presumably function) occur (Pantelis et al 2003). This might herald the beginning of further neurobiological changes as the disorder progresses. What is unclear is when exactly these changes begin, whether they can be prevented, reversed or modified in some way with intervention and whether there is a point at which irreversible brain damage has occurred and chronic psychotic disorder is inevitable.

The fact that a considerable amount of psychiatric symptoms, disability, and self-harming and other health-damaging behaviours occur during this prodromal phase (Yung and Jackson 1999; Yung et al 2003, in press) and this

more recent research suggesting some neurobiological change during the prodrome have been the impetus for renewed efforts at attempting to intervene at this early stage. If the prodrome can be recognized prospectively and treatment provided at this stage, then disability could be minimized, some recovery may be possible before symptoms and poor functioning become entrenched and the possibility of preventing, delaying or ameliorating the onset of diagnosable psychotic disorder arises. Neurobiological changes that occur around the time of onset of full blown psychotic disorder could also be prevented, minimized or reversed.

It is speculated that young people experiencing this early phase of illness might engage more quickly with treatment than young people who are acutely unwell and possibly experiencing symptoms that deter them from seeking assistance and support. If the 'prodromal' young people do become more unwell, the need for hospitalization might be reduced because effective treatment can be provided rapidly, without delay. Similarly, they might be more likely to accept treatment if acute psychosis does emerge than young people who have been acutely unwell for considerably longer before assistance is sought.

Other benefits of pre-psychotic intervention include the capacity to research the onset phase of illness and examine the psychobiology of progression from the subthreshold state to the fully fledged disorder. More proximal risk factors, such as substance use, stress and the underlying neurobiology, can also be uniquely studied. The delineation of this discrete phase, the boundaries of which are often difficult to map precisely, is of great heuristic and practical value. Box 2.1 summarizes the key reasons for attempting some form of pre-psychotic intervention.

Box 2.1
Potential advantages of pre-psychotic intervention[1]

- The onset of psychosis may be prevented. This would represent a reduction in incidence of full blown psychotic disorder.
- Neurobiological changes that may occur around the time of psychosis onset could also be prevented or minimized.
- The onset of psychosis could be ameliorated. Thus, hospitalization and other lifestyle disruption would be minimized, and as psychotic symptoms are less likely to be entrenched, then management of the disorder could be made easier and more effective.
- The onset of psychosis could be delayed. This might result in marked reductions in morbidity and a consequent fall in both the human and economic costs of the disorder. The impact of a first episode of psychosis on a 16-year-old is likely to adversely effect personality development, self-esteem, significant relationships, educational attainment and vocational trajectory much more so than if the first episode occurred in a 30-year-old. This opinion is supported by the fact that the outcome for adolescents with early onset schizophrenia is significantly worse than that for those with an onset in middle to late adult life (Krausz and Muller-Thomsen 1993). Even the deferment of psychosis by one year without any lessening of subsequent morbidity would dramatically reduce the costs of treating the disorder (McGorry et al 2001).
- An avenue for help is provided, irrespective of whether transition to psychotic disorder ultimately occurs, to tackle the serious problems of social withdrawal, impaired functioning and subjective distress that might otherwise become entrenched and steadily worsen.
- Young people who attend the service are provided with support and assistance targeted at other issues and problems they might be experiencing, including mental health issues, such as depression, anxiety disorders or substance use. This intervention might prevent, delay or ameliorate other mental health disorders that might otherwise have developed.
- Engagement and trust are easier to develop and thus a foundation is laid for later therapeutic interventions, especially drug therapy if and when required. The family can be similarly engaged and provided with emotional support and information outside of a highly charged crisis situation.
- If psychosis develops, it can be detected rapidly and duration of untreated psychosis minimized. This is important as prolonged duration of untreated psychosis has been found to be a predictor of poor outcome of schizophrenia.
- If psychosis develops then treatment can be commenced in a timely and non-traumatic manner. A crisis with behavioural disturbance or self-harm is not required to gain access to treatment.
- Comorbidity, such as depression and substance abuse, can be effectively treated and the patient therefore gets immediate benefits
- The prospective study of the transition process is enabled, including neurobiological, psychopathological and environmental aspects. Patients are less impaired cognitively and emotionally and are more likely to be fully competent to give informed consent for such research endeavours.

[1] Adapted from McGorry PD, Yung AR, Phillips LJ (2003). The 'close-in' or ultra high risk model: A safe and effective strategy for research and clinical intervention in prepsychotic mental disorder. *Schizophr Bull* 29: 771–790.

Consequently, pre-psychotic or 'prodromal' intervention has a dual focus: (1) treatment of the symptoms and disability that the individual is experiencing currently; and (2) the prevention of full-blown disorder. It is therefore an example of what has been termed 'indicated prevention'.

Intervention in the psychotic 'prodrome'—the indicated prevention model

Interventions can be broadly classified as prevention, treatment and maintenance. Within prevention, three subclassifications of interventions have been described: universal, selective and indicated (Gordon 1983; Mrazek and Haggarty 1994). *Universal* preventive interventions are targeted to the general public or a whole population group that has not been identified on the basis of individual risk. Promotion of the use of seat belts, immunization, and non-smoking policies are all examples of universal prevention approaches. *Selective* preventive measures are appropriate for subgroups of the population whose risk of becoming ill is above average. Examples include special immunizations, such as travellers to areas where yellow fever is endemic and annual mammograms for women with a positive family history of breast cancer. The subjects are clearly asymptomatic. This has been the level of prevention underpinning the traditional genetic high risk studies in schizophrenia which have identified people at risk solely on the basis of family history of schizophrenia (see Asarnow 1988 for a review). In contrast, *indicated* preventive measures apply to those individuals who on examination are found to manifest a risk factor that identifies them, *individually*, as being at high risk for the future development of a disease, and as such could be the focus of screening.

Within the mental health field, indicated prevention is:

> ...*targeted to high-risk individuals who are identified as having minimal but detectable signs or symptoms foreshadowing mental disorder, or biological markers indicating predisposition for mental disorder, but who do not meet... diagnostic levels at the current time.*
> (Mrazek and Haggarty 1994, p 154)

Thus, indicated prevention focuses on people with early and/or subthreshold features of mental disorder. That is, they are symptomatic: already experiencing a degree of suffering and disability.

Summary

- A significant degree of the disability and functional decline associated with psychotic disorders emerges during the prodromal phase of illness prior to the onset of frank psychotic symptoms.
- It has been speculated that the level of functional decline associated with the prodrome might create a ceiling for eventual recovery in young people with psychotic disorders.
- If psychotic prodromes can be recognized and intervention provided at this early stage, then onset of psychotic disorder may be prevented, ameliorated or delayed.
- Additionally, duration of untreated psychosis can be minimized for those people who do develop a psychotic disorder, research into this crucial phase can be undertaken and factors which increase or decrease the likelihood of transition to full blown psychotic disorder can be studied.

Given its potential importance, the conceptual underpinnings of pre-psychotic intervention need to be considered. The concept of the prodrome in psychotic disorders, the distinction between the prodrome and the premorbid phase, and between the prodrome and frank psychosis need to be elucidated. These issues are highlighted in the following chapter.

References

Agerbo E, Byrne M, Eaton WW, Mortensen PB (2003). Schizophrenia, marital status and employment: A forty year study. *Schizophr Res* **60**(suppl):32.

Asarnow JR (1988) Children at risk for schizophrenia: Converging lines of evidence. *Schizophr Bull* **14**:613–630.

Done DJ, Crow TJ, Johnstone EC, Sacker A. (1994) Childhood antecedents of schizophrenia and affective illness: social adjustment at ages 7 and 11. *BMJ* **309**:699–703.

Fava GA, Kellner R (1991) Prodromal symptoms in affective disorders. *Am J Psychiatry* **148**:823–830.

Gordon RS (1983) An operational classification of disease prevention. *Public Health Rep* **98**:107–109.

Häfner H, Nowotny B, Loffler W, et al (1995). When and how does schizophrenia produce social deficits? *Eur Arch Psychiatry Clin Neurosci* **246**:17–28.

Jones P, Rodgers B, Murray R, Marmot M (1994) Child development risk factors for adult schizophrenia in the British 1946 birth cohort. *Lancet* **344**:1398–1402.

Krausz M, Muller-Thomsen TSO (1993) Schizophrenia with onset in adolescence: An 11-year follow up. *Schizophr Bull* **19**:831–841.

McGorry PD, Yung AR, Phillips LJ (2001) 'Closing in': What features predict the onset of first episode psychosis within a high risk group? In Zipursky RB,

Schulz SC, eds, *The early stages of schizophrenia*. Washington DC: American Psychiatric Press: 3–32.

McGorry PD, Yung AR, Phillips LJ (2003) The 'close-in' or ultra high risk model: A safe and effective strategy for research and clinical intervention in prepsychotic mental disorder. *Schizophr Bull* **29**: 771–790.

Meares A (1959) The diagnosis of prepsychotic schizophrenia. *Lancet* **I**:55–59.

Mrazek PJ, Haggarty RJ (1994) *Reducing risks for mental disorders: Frontiers for preventive intervention research*. Washington DC: National Academy Press.

Pantelis C, Velakoulis D, McGorry PD, et al (2003) Neuroanatomical abnormalities before and after onset of psychosis: A cross-sectional and longitudinal MRI comparison. *Lancet* **361**:281–288.

Post SG (2001) Preventing schizophrenia and Alzheimer disease: Comparative ethics. *Schizophr Res* **51**:103–108.

Sullivan HS (1927, reprinted 1994) The onset of schizophrenia. *Am J Psychiatry* **151**:135–139.

Yung AR, McGorry PD (1996) The prodromal phase of first-episode psychosis: Past and current conceptualizations. *Schizophr Bull* **22**:353–370.

Yung AR, Jackson HJ (1999) The onset of psychotic disorder: Clinical and research aspects. In McGorry PD, Jackson HJ, eds, *The recognition and management of early psychosis: A preventive approach*. Cambridge University Press: 27–50.

Yung AR, Phillips LJ, Yuen HP, et al (2003) Psychosis prediction: 12 month follow-up of a high risk ('prodromal') group. *Schizophr Res* **60**:21–32.

Yung AR, Phillips LJ, Yuen HP, McGorry PD (in press) Risk factors for psychosis: Psychopathology and clinical features. *Schizophr Res.*

Conceptual and background issues

3

The concept of the prodrome in psychotic disorders

As noted previously, the 'prodrome' is a term used in clinical medicine to refer to the early symptoms and signs that a person experiences before the full-blown syndrome of an illness becomes evident. We have previously used the example of the disease measles to illustrate this point. Measles is characterized by a three to four day prodromal period of fever, cough, coryza and conjunctivitis, followed by the development of the distinctive rash (Yung et al 2001). This is a neat example, with a clear-cut onset and offset of the prodrome and the definitive disorder itself.

An example from clinical medicine with a more diffuse pattern, which more closely parallels the situation in psychotic disorders, is that of hepatitis A. This disease usually begins with a non-specific prodrome of fever, aches and pains, anorexia and loss of taste for food and cigarettes. A definitive diagnosis of a hepatitis syndrome is made after the appearance of clinical jaundice and serological tests. The latter also identify the specific subtype of hepatitis that is present (Elias 1983). However, more subtle signs of impending hepatitis can be detected by the astute clinician prior to the appearance of frank jaundice, such as dark urine or a slight tinge of yellow colour in the sclera. Thus, the definitive sign of disease (clinical jaundice) differs qualitatively from the non-specific prodromal features (fever, aches and pains), and differs quantitatively from early subtle forms of jaundice (Elias 1983).

An analogy can be drawn here with psychotic disorders, which are usually preceded by a non-specific prodromal period. For example, depressed mood, anxiety and irritability commonly precede a first psychotic episode (Yung and McGorry 1996). The definitive psychotic symptoms occur later and a diagnosis of psychotic disorder can be made when they worsen. This diagnosis could be schizophrenia, schizophreniform disorder, bipolar disorder with psychotic features, or any other psychotic disorder. However, subtle 'attenuated' forms of psychotic symptoms, are likely to have been present prior to the psychotic symptoms being obvious—possibly during the period of anxiety and depression—just as a subtle form of jaundice would have present prior to clinical jaundice being obvious. These subthreshold psychotic symptoms deviate from normal phenomena but are not frankly psychotic. Examples include overvalued ideas that people are laughing at or are hostile towards the person, but the person realizes that it is not really true and that he or she is just being 'a bit paranoid'. A strange feeling of change in the self, others or the world in the absence of any crystallized delusion is another example. Perceptual disturbances, too, can occur in forms that are not clear hallucinations, that is, they are below psychotic intensity, such as visual or auditory distortions. Thus, the difference between these phenomena and frank psychotic symptoms is in the degree or intensity of the symptom. These types of phenomena have been described in retrospective studies of emerging first episode psychosis or psychotic relapse (Møller and Husby 2000; Yung and McGorry 1996, 1997).

Hence, from a symptomatic view, it seems that the non-specific prodromal features (depressed mood and so on) differ qualitatively from the definitive clinical syndrome (psychosis), but that the definitive syndrome is also preceded by features that differ from it only quantitatively (attenuated psychotic symptoms).

Thus two related questions arise. (1) How should the beginning of *illness* be defined? The crux of this question is determining the boundary between premorbid state and onset of illness. Hence, the issue of distinguishing 'normality' from 'abnormality' becomes relevant. This question could be reframed as the determination of the onset of the prodrome. (2) When does a *prodrome* end and the *definitive disorder* begin? At the heart of this question is defining the onset of psychosis. These two questions will be considered in turn.

Defining the onset of the prodrome

Prodrome is a retrospective concept

Reverting to the hepatitis analogy, just as the fever, aches and pains are considered, in retrospect, to be part of the hepatitis disease itself, the depression, anxiety and irritability could be considered, in retrospect, to be part of the psychotic disorder itself. The important caveat included in these statements is that this diagnostic process occurs *in retrospect*. This is true not only in psychiatry but clinical medicine as well. A clinical picture of fever, aches and pains cannot be diagnosed clinically as hepatitis. Any one of a number of illnesses may eventually develop, or the syndrome may resolve without any definitive diagnosis being made. Similarly, one cannot 'diagnose' a psychotic prodrome (ie impending psychotic disorder) with any certainty based on the presence of, for example, depression, anxiety and social isolation. These symptoms may indicate the presence of a threshold or subthreshold mood disorder, substance use, a physical illness or simply a reaction to circumstances. A first episode of psychosis cannot even be predicted from the presence of attenuated psychotic symptoms as these symptoms, also, can resolve before a full-blown psychotic disorder develops. This has been observed on numerous occasions in our patient population (see Case Study 1).

Case Study 1: Lucia

Lucia was a 17-year-old student in her final year at high school. She was referred to the PACE Clinic by a psychologist at her school who had spoken with Lucia at the request of her teachers who were concerned about changes in her behaviour. They had noticed that she had become distant from most of her friends and had uncharacteristically become verbally abusive towards one of them, accusing her of talking about her behind her back. The school psychologist consulted with Lucia's parents who indicated that Lucia was spending more time in her bedroom alone recently. Lucia said that over the past three months she had developed ideas that her family and friends were conspiring to harm her in some way. She said that she knew that this could not be true but was avoiding contact with others because this reduced the frequency of these thoughts. She indicated that on about four occasions in the past month she had had experiences of hearing mumbling voices outside her head. On two occasions, these experiences occurred as she was trying to get to sleep

and on another occasion the voices were clearer and were speaking negatively about her. Lucia expressed concern at these experiences and relief that she was able to speak about them with somebody.

Lucia was assessed at the PACE Clinic. She said that she had experienced similar symptoms on and off for the past eighteen months—usually coinciding with increased stressors in her life. Indeed, she spoke of feeling anxious about her forthcoming exams and concerns that she would not achieve high enough marks to be able to commence the university degree she was interested in the following year. Lucia noted that her symptoms usually abated as the stressor passed. Indeed, speaking about her concerns and learning some stress reduction strategies, Lucia indicated that the symptoms reduced in frequency and intensity.

After three months, these experiences had abated.

Further evidence indicating that attenuated psychotic symptoms do not inevitably evolve into a full-blown psychotic disorder lies in the finding that these attenuated psychotic symptoms and 'psychotic-like experiences' are not uncommonly found in the general population, at far higher rates than psychotic disorders (Peters 2001; Peters et al 1999; van Os et al 2000, 2001). This indicates that at least some attenuated psychotic symptoms must either resolve without full-blown psychosis ensuing or that they can persist without developing into a full-blown psychotic disorder.

Distinguishing 'normal' from 'abnormal'

This issue of distinguishing 'normal' from 'abnormal' needs to be addressed if we are to answer the question about the onset of prodromes. The finding of high levels of attenuated psychotic symptoms and 'psychotic-like experiences' in the general population (Peters et al 1999; van Os et al 2001) has important implications for defining this boundary.

Some parallels can again be drawn with hepatitis (the psychotic disorder equivalent) and subtle jaundice (the attenuated psychotic symptoms equivalent). Some people can develop subtle jaundice that is not noticed by others and for which they do not seek help. This can spontaneously resolve without ever developing into clinical hepatitis. Others can have other diseases (such as Gilbert's disease), causing them to be mildly jaundiced intermittently in response to acute intercurrent infections, such as the common cold or other stressors. They usually do not seek medical treatment for the jaundice, which remits when the acute condition resolves. Some other clinical conditions, such as Crigler-

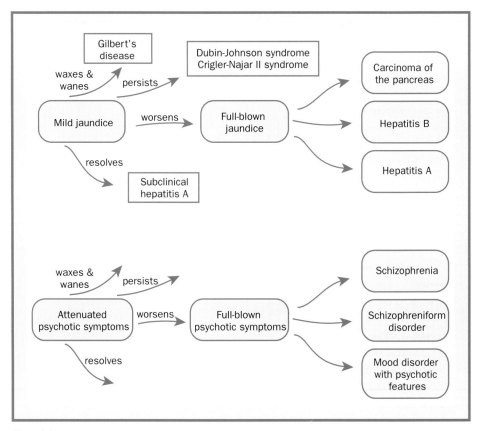

Figure 3.1
Parallels between the syndrome of mild jaundice and its range of outcomes, with the syndrome of attenuated psychotic symptoms and its range of outcomes

Najar syndrome type II and Dubin-Johnson syndrome, can cause chronic mild jaundice for which the individual may never seek treatment (Elias 1983). Thus, the clinical syndrome of jaundice has several different underlying causes. Equally, jaundice can follow a number of clinical courses. In some cases, the course can be benign, rarely leading to help-seeking, liver impairment or premature death. This is the case with Gilbert's disease. Other cases of jaundice can occasionally have a benign course but at other times can be more severe. Finally, some cases of jaundice may usually or inevitably be associated with liver impairment, overt symptoms of liver failure and premature death (eg carcinoma of the head of the pancreas: Elias 1983).

In the same way, we hypothesize that attenuated psychotic symptoms can follow a number of courses. They can occur then resolve spontaneously without any treatment-seeking, they can occur intermittently, perhaps in response to some stressor, or they can be present chronically but without resulting in distress or help-seeking, in addition to the possibility that they can worsen and develop into a full-blown psychotic disorder. As with the jaundice analogy, attenuated psychotic symptoms make up a clinical syndrome that may have multiple underlying etiologies, all with different likelihoods of causing functional impairment, distress and help-seeking. Figure 3.1 illustrates the parallels between jaundice and psychosis.

Community studies are consistent with this theory (Eaton et al 1989; van Os et al 2001) but more research is needed to investigate whether the different course and outcomes of attenuated psychotic symptoms are etiologically distinct from each other. What would be useful would be to discover if benign forms of attenuated psychotic symptoms can be distinguished from

those symptoms that presage high likelihood of development of full-blown psychotic disorder.

Defining the onset of psychosis

Many studies have attempted to define the onset of psychosis retrospectively in established psychotic disorders such as schizophrenia. There are several difficulties in establishing this time point, such as uncertainty about which types of symptoms should be used to define psychosis (the definition could be restricted to hallucinations and delusions or could include disorganized speech and behaviour as well), and deciding when the symptom has become sufficiently deviant to be labelled psychotic. The subjective nature of psychotic symptoms also needs to be considered—observers often date onset of psychotic symptoms well after the individual recalls them beginning (Häfner et al 1993; Norman and Malla 2001; Yung and McGorry 1996).

Structured and semi-structured instruments are currently available for the retrospective assessment of onset of psychosis, including the Royal Park Multidiagnostic Instrument for Psychosis (RPMIP: McGorry et al 1990a, b), the Interview for the Retrospective Assessment of the Onset of Schizophrenia (IRAOS: Häfner et al 1992) and the Comprehensive Assessment of Symptoms and History (CASH: Andreasen et al 1992). Each of these instruments has their own standardized approaches, with arbitrary decisions about when to date timing of onset of disorder. However, even such standardized approaches are not immune from potential sources of inaccuracy, such as recall bias and 'effort after meaning', a situation that may arise when the patient or family wish to attribute the onset of illness to a particular precipitating event (eg 'it all started after I hit my head on the mantelpiece') (Yung and McGorry 1996).

Psychotic symptoms rarely arise suddenly, but are more likely to gradually evolve and worsen, from an attenuated state to a full threshold state. Most clinicians have no difficulty in diagnosing a full-blown psychotic syndrome in a patient, but more subtle early psychotic features may be more difficult to recognize. Box 3.1 summarizes some of the reasons why recognizing the onset of psychosis prospectively is not always clear-cut.

Indeed, in a recent large epidemiological study of psychotic and psychotic-like phenomena, symptoms that were described as 'plausible' (having some possible explanation) by lay interviewers were strongly associated with actual psychotic symptoms as rated by a psychiatrist (odds ratio 11.4–22.0: van Os et al 2000). Furthermore, young people experiencing psychotic symptoms for the first time may lack awareness that the phenomena they are experiencing are the products of a mental illness and this may delay them reporting such experiences to others (Thompson et al 2001). They also rarely have the terminology to describe such events (Thompson et al 2001). For example, rather than saying that they hear 'voices' young people might report intrusive thoughts, or use other descriptions. Case Studies 2 and 3 illustrate some of these points related to defining onset of psychosis.

Case Study 2: Mehmet
Mehmet was a 19-year-old university student studying information technology. He had been shy all his life, but found himself becoming increasingly self-conscious to the extent that he eventually believed that others were looking at him.

Box 3.1
Defining the onset of psychosis prospectively—situations that complicate the definition

---

Gradual onset
- of symptoms, especially symptoms which seem to evolve out of underlying personality

Fluctuations
- in intensity and frequency of the symptoms
- in level of insight into the symptoms

Appraisal of the symptoms
- individual may not be aware that the experiences are unusual or abnormal
- individual may attribute them to a variety of sources, some plausible
- observers may attribute the symptoms to a range of plausible explanations
- one individual may not be distressed by the same type of symptoms that another would be disturbed by

Lack of terminology
- individual may not have the language to describe the phenomena

Variability in the impact of the symptoms
- individual may not be disabled by or seek help for the symptoms

He became unable to attend tutorials as he felt that others in the class thought he was stupid. He became so preoccupied with these concerns that he could no longer concentrate in lectures or on his studies at home. He then started to think that other students would know that he had fallen behind in his work. He gradually developed more and more negative interpretations of actual and perceived attention, such as when anyone looked at him in the street he would think they were thinking he was stupid. Finally, he formed frank persecutory beliefs that others, even strangers, knew he was failing his course and that he was a useless person. These thoughts fluctuated in intensity and frequency at first before becoming continuous and persistently delusional.

Case Study 3: Belinda

Belinda was a 21-year-old single office worker who described having loud thoughts in her head ever since childhood. At first, these thoughts were her own thoughts and under her control, and it felt like she could have conversations with herself in her head. She had not thought this abnormal until there was a gradual change in their quality when she was about 15. They became more intrusive, sometimes keeping her awake at night, although she still recognized them as her own thoughts. She started to notice that at times of stress they would be particularly intense and could sometimes feel like they were coming from outside her head as well as from within it. They then also seemed to take on a more alien quality, not always seeming like her own thoughts, but initially this waxed and waned. She sought help because the experiences, which she sometimes described as 'thoughts' and sometimes as 'voices', began to interfere with her work. They also started telling her that her work colleagues did not like her and she became distressed by this. Eventually, she developed nearly continuous auditory hallucinations and persecutory delusions involving her colleagues.

Another issue that makes the prospective diagnosis of first episode psychosis challenging is that of the definition of psychotic disorder or disorders and how they relate to psychotic symptoms *per se*. Does the mere presence of a psychotic *symptom* mean that the person has a psychotic *disorder*? Again, referring to the general population studies previously cited (Peters 2001; Peters et al 1999; van Os et al 1999, 2000), it is clear that a substantial minority of people in the community experience psychotic symptoms at some point in their lives, and they are not invariably distressed by them. Should they be considered to have a disorder? Or should disorder only be diagnosed in the presence of impaired functioning, disability, help-seeking and/or distress? The level of intensity of psychotic symptoms, their frequency and duration also need to be factored into the definition. Is there an absolute level of intensity, frequency and duration of symptoms considered to be at acute psychotic threshold? Or should different levels of symptoms be applied depending on variables, such as distress and disability? Other parameters that could be included in a definition of psychotic 'disorder' include presence or absence and degree of comorbidity with other psychiatric syndromes, such as depression, and level of suicidality and dangerousness.

These issues are yet to be resolved. Indeed, any further discussion about the definition of psychotic disorder is likely to become embroiled in debate about the definition of health, disease and illness in general, a subject which can only be touched upon here. A major source of disagreement about defining these concepts is the role of values and value judgements in making decisions about presence or absence of health and disease (Campbell et al 1979; Fulford 2001; Perring 2001; Scadding 1990). Psychiatry is rife with value judgements being used to define disorder. For example, the Introductions of the third edition (revised) and fourth edition of the Diagnostic and Statistical Manual for Mental Disorders (DSM) state that the presence of a *clinically significant* behavioural or psychological syndrome is required to diagnose a mental disorder (American Psychiatric Association 1987, 1994). But such a description requires someone to make a judgement about clinical significance. To make this decision, various value judgements are needed, for instance about the quality of the person's relationships, their use of time, their educational and vocational achievements, and so on. Some have distinguished between 'disease' and 'illness' by conceptualizing disease as an 'underlying (value-free) process, which is only transformed into illness if it is serious enough to be incapacitating and therefore undesirable to its bearer' (Boorse

1975, p 61). Similar is the statement that 'disease/illness are conditions people suffer that need to be defined because they want them treated' (Kottow 2002, p 79). However, both these definitions are problematic when applied to psychiatry, particularly in relation to the psychoses. Patients with psychotic disorders, such as schizophrenia, may well be incapacitated and suffering but do not necessarily see their condition as undesirable or in need of treatment. Thus, such definitions do not really help us when considering what parameters should be included in a definition of psychosis, particularly when the boundaries with normality are concerned. How deviant from 'normal thinking' or 'normal behaviour or functioning' does a symptom or behaviour need to be to be accepted as indicative of disease or disorder?

What is needed is some evidence base for making these decisions. The essence of any psychiatric disorder should be that it is associated with some distress or impairment in functioning, or with some adverse outcome, for instance problems in long-term functioning. Both terms these criteria are of course value-laden.

We do know that the community-based studies have found that those who seek help for attenuated and frank psychotic symptoms have much higher levels of distress when compared to non-help-seekers, and comorbid disorders, particularly depression. Furthermore, psychotic experiences accompanied by distress and help-seeking were significantly more likely to predict future clinical need than those without distress or help-seeking (Hanssen et al submitted). Community studies also suggest that isolated and/or attenuated psychotic symptoms: (a) are associated with decreased quality of life, even when the symptoms are not distressing (van Os et al 2001), and (b) are associated with increased risk of developing full-blown psychotic disorders in the future (Poulton et al 2000). If the essence of defining a disorder lies in it requiring treatment of some kind, then it would seem that dimensions such as these (functioning, disability, help-seeking and/or distress) should be incorporated into any definition of psychotic disorder. This is, however, not currently the case in the DSM system (American Psychiatric Association 1994), under which it is possible to diagnose schizophreniform disorder, brief psychotic disorder, substance-induced psychotic disorder and psychotic disorder not otherwise specified by the presence of psychotic symptoms alone without the requirement of any associated functional impact or disability. In fact, schizophrenia is the only psychotic disorder that requires a criterion of psychosocial impairment.

At this stage, we have chosen to operationalize a definition of psychosis based on the presence of clear-cut threshold level psychotic symptoms (delusions, hallucinations and formal thought disorder) occurring several times per week for at least one week (see Box 3.2) in a help-seeking population.

This threshold is essentially that at which neuroleptic medication would be commenced in common clinical practice and was developed via

Box 3.2
Definition of psychosis onset

- Psychotic symptoms. Presence of at least one of the following: ideas of reference, magical thinking, perceptual disturbance, paranoid ideation, odd thinking and speech.
- Duration of episode of greater than one week.
- Frequency of symptoms. At least several times per week.

local consensus of psychiatrists at PACE and EPPIC (McGorry et al 1996) in Melbourne, Australia. This definition of onset of psychosis is, of course, somewhat arbitrary, but does at least have clear treatment implications and applies equally well to substance-related symptoms, symptoms that have a mood component—either depression or mania—and schizophrenia spectrum disorders. However, it does not include a requirement of functional impairment or decline. This is an area currently under consideration in our Clinic. This highlights the arbitrariness of any operational definition, which is inherently open to error, and emphasizes that all such definitions must continually be reviewed. Case Study 4 illustrates the process of onset of psychotic disorder. This can be gradual, with an evolving pattern of symptom acquisition and intensification and with fluctuations in severity.

Case Study 4: Andrew
Andrew was a 25-year-old single man studying law at university. He described about a two year history of feeling fatigued and irritable and said it had been increasingly difficult for him to attend his course and complete his assignments over the last six months. He found he could not concentrate properly and had difficulty remembering. He had been feeling annoyed with his family for no reason and decided he did not like anyone. He stopped seeing his friends over the last six months. About three months prior to being admitted to hospital he developed occasional strange tastes in his mouth, and a few weeks prior

to admission had 'realized' that his mother had been poisoning him. He stated that this was the cause of his concentration and memory problems. He was hospitalized after he attacked his mother.

Characterizing the prodrome

Symptoms and signs

If psychotic prodromes are to be recognized, there must be some characterization of the symptoms and signs of this phase. Several researchers have examined the issue of which features are characteristic of the psychotic prodrome. The literature varies in approach and extent. Some studies have made detailed retrospective descriptions of the symptoms and signs leading up to a first episode of either psychosis as a syndrome (Yung and McGorry 1996) or schizophrenia as a specific diagnosis. The epidemiological papers of Häfner's group in Germany are an example of this, and are particularly sound as data were collected using the standardized structured instrument mentioned earlier— the IRAOS (Häfner et al 1992) using a large sample size. However, this method is extremely time-consuming

A different approach is to prospectively follow-up patients with already diagnosed schizophrenia and examine the prodromal features leading up to a psychotic relapse. Thus, the *relapse prodrome* rather than the *initial prodrome* is the subject of investigation in these studies. In some studies of relapse prodrome antipsychotic medication is ceased in order to observe emerging psychosis (Donlon and Blacker

1973) and others follow a more naturalistic design (Birchwood et al 1989; Heinrichs and Carpenter 1985; Subotnik and Nuechterlein 1988). The problem with this method is that it has not been established how the signs and symptoms of a relapse prodrome in schizophrenia relate to the prodromal features of a first psychotic episode. Some symptoms may be modified by such factors as medication, the fear of relapse and hospitalization, and the family's changing perception of the patient. In fact, in one study of relapse prodrome, concern about the possibility of relapse is mentioned as an early symptom by patients who were taken off maintenance medication and observed (Donlon and Blacker 1973).

Box 3.3 summarizes this existing literature accumulated on schizophrenic prodromes, indicating the most commonly described prodromal features.

As can be seen, the most frequently occurring prodromal features are non-specific: reduced concentration and attention, decreased

Box 3.3
Most frequent prodromal symptoms described in retrospective studies[1]

- Reduced concentration and attention
- Reduced drive and motivation
- Depression
- Sleep disturbance
- Anxiety
- Social withdrawal
- Suspiciousness
- Deterioration in role functioning
- Irritability

[1]Adapted from Yung AR, McGorry PD (1996) The prodromal phase of first-episode psychosis: Past and current conceptualizations. *Schizophr Bull* **22**: 353-370.

motivation, sleep disturbance, depressed mood and anxiety. However, suspiciousness, an attenuated form of persecutory delusions, and other attenuated or subthreshold psychotic symptoms are also frequently reported. This list obviously does not cover the full range of prodromal symptoms described in the various studies. These are summarized in Table 3.1, and the reader is referred to the paper by Yung and McGorry (1996) for a comprehensive list of the studies which described these various features. Essentially, they can be divided into eight main subtypes: (1) neurotic symptoms; (2) mood-related symptoms; (3) changes in volition; (4) cognitive changes; (5) physical symptoms; (6) attenuated or subthreshold versions of psychotic symptoms; (7) other symptoms; and (8) behavioural changes.

Another important body of literature relevant to the characterization and conceptualization of the initial psychotic prodrome is that of Huber and colleagues from Bonn, Germany. They propose that the earliest manifestations of schizophrenia are 'basic symptoms'—subjectively experienced abnormalities in the realms of cognition, attention, perception and movement. Also described as 'self-experienced neuropsychological deficits' (Klosterkötter et al 1996), these basic symptoms are different from Bleulerian fundamental symptoms and their modern operationalized successors, the negative symptoms (Klosterkötter et al 1996). Negative symptoms are externally observed by others, but basic symptoms can only be subjectively identified by the person experiencing them. However, there may be a continuum with some basic symptoms being the precursors to the objectively observed negative symptoms.

The basic symptoms are numerous, and detailed descriptions can be found in Gross and

Table 3.1
Prodromal features of schizophrenia

1. Neurotic symptoms
   - Anxiety
   - Restlessness
   - Anger, irritability

2. Mood-related symptoms
   - Depression
   - Anhedonia
   - Guilt
   - Suicidal ideas
   - Mood swings

3. Changes in volition
   - Apathy, loss of drive
   - Boredom, loss of interest
   - Fatigue, reduced energy

4. Cognitive changes
   - Disturbance of attention and concentration
   - Preoccupation, daydreaming
   - Thought-blocking
   - Reduced abstraction

5. Physical symptoms
   - Somatic complaints
   - Loss of weight
   - Poor appetite
   - Sleep disturbance

6. Attenuated or subthreshold versions of psychotic symptoms
   - Perceptual abnormalities
   - Suspiciousness
   - Change in sense of self, others or the world
   - Change in affect
   - Change in motility

7. Other symptoms
   - Obsessive-compulsive phenomena
   - Dissociative phenomena
   - Increased interpersonal sensitivity

8. Behavioural changes
   - Deterioration in role-functioning
   - Social withdrawal
   - Impulsivity
   - Odd behaviour
   - Aggressive, disruptive behaviour

Huber 1996, Klosterkötter et al 1996 and the semi-structured interview schedule specifically designed to assess them, the Bonn Scale for Assessment of Basic Symptoms (BSABS: Klosterkötter et al 1997). They include: (1) disorders of drive, such as increased fatigability and decreased energy; (2) disorders of stress tolerance including impaired ability to cope with unusual or unexpected demands and inability to work under pressure; (3) disorders of affect and emotional reactivity, such as reduced capacity to discriminate between different kinds of emotions and decrease in the need for contact with others; (4) cognitive disorders, such as thought blockages, and problems with concentration and memory; (5) perceptual disturbances, such as distortions, illusions and hypersensitivity to light and noise; (6) motor disorders, such as subjectively experienced disturbances of movement; and (7) impaired or unusual bodily sensations, termed *cenesthesias*, including sensations of movement, pulling or pressure inside the body or on its surface, and sensations of the body or parts of it extending, diminishing, shrinking, enlarging, growing or constricting (Klosterkötter et al 1997).

The Bonn group have subclassified basic symptoms into 'level 1' and 'level 2' symptoms. Level 1 basic symptoms are described as 'uncharacteristic' or non-specific, that is, they can occur in other psychiatric disorders (Gross and Huber 1996). Level 2 basic symptoms have been called 'rather characteristic', meaning that they are more often seen in schizophrenia than non-psychotic disorders (Gross and Huber 1996). In fact, the level 1 basic symptoms are rather like the non-specific prodromal symptoms previously described (anxiety and depression, for example), although the basic symptoms are described in much more detail and emphasize

the subjective nature of the disturbances. The Bonn group note that the level 1 basic symptoms are the earliest manifestations of the psychotic prodrome and are frequently diagnosed as anxiety, somatoform or personality disorders according to traditional Anglophone classificatory systems such as the DSM (American Psychiatric Association 1994). Some of the level 2 basic symptoms are objectively observable and known in the Anglophone literature as 'negative symptoms'. Other level 2 basic symptoms are forms of attenuated psychotic symptoms, such as perceptual abnormalities and various forms of overvalued ideas.

Pattern of the prodrome

The most commonly described pattern of prodromal symptoms is that of a gradual onset beginning with non-specific neurotic-type symptoms followed by the usually slow development of unusual ideas (eg suspiciousness), or vague ideas of reference, and finally the development of frank psychotic symptoms. Symptoms are at first mainly subjective and not detectable by others (Yung and McGorry 1996). Eventually, they become more severe and are usually accompanied by some deterioration in role-functioning and other behavioural changes (Bowers 1965; Cameron 1938; Chapman and Chapman 1987; Docherty et al 1978; Donlon and Blacker 1973; Heinrichs and Carpenter 1985; Herz and Melville 1980; Meares 1959). Fluctuations in symptoms can occur, not necessarily in relation to any particular trigger or change in circumstance. Frank delusions often 'crystallize' out of previously vague feelings of something being not right. The 'crystallization' occurs when the individual forms an explanatory model for the unusual experiences that have been affecting him or her (Cameron 1938). The primary abnormality is commonly a disturbance of perception or cognition.

The basic symptoms theorists have a similar model for understanding the process of onset of psychosis. They suggest that the development of clinical schizophrenia follows a sequence of events beginning with the level 1 basic symptoms, followed by the level 2 basic symptoms, and finally the development of positive symptoms. The change from level 1 to level 2 occurs when the person experiences their deficiencies as being more strange, irritation increases and dismay develops. For example, the person may feel 'as if' thoughts are being interfered with or influenced from the outside. As the intensity of these symptoms worsens, the 'as if' component becomes overwhelmed, and the final 'crystallization' into delusions of thought insertion, thought withdrawal and/or thought broadcasting occurs when the person works out 'how', 'why' and 'by whom' the interference with his or her thoughts has taken place (Klosterkötter 1992). Thus, the proponents of basic symptoms hypothesize that positive psychotic symptoms emerge from their basic symptom precursors. Other examples include thought withdrawal arising from feelings of blocked thoughts and somatic hallucinations evolving from cenesthesias (altered bodily sensations: Gross and Huber 1996).

As noted in relation to non-specific prodromal symptoms and attenuated psychotic symptoms, basic symptoms are said to fluctuate in severity and occurrence. Endogenous variations occur as well as variations in response to stress (Gross and Huber 1996).

Duration of the prodrome

Retrospective studies suggest that virtually all patients experience a prodromal phase, which varies in duration from a very brief period to several years. Some have suggested that the duration of the average prodrome has a bimodal distribution, less than one year for some patients and over four years for others (Varsamis and Adamson 1971). Other retrospective studies have described the prodromes as variable in length, ranging from 0, that is, no prodrome at all, to 20 years (Beiser et al 1993). Loebel and colleagues found that the time interval from the onset of prodromal symptoms to the onset of psychotic symptoms was a mean of 98.5 weeks (Loebel et al 1992). This time interval was not significantly different for schizophrenic and schizoaffective subjects. There was no significant gender difference.

Thus, the research findings suggest that the duration of the prodrome before the first episode of psychosis in schizophrenia is often prolonged, up to several years. In contrast, prodromal symptoms preceding psychotic relapse have been found to be much briefer in duration, around 2–4 weeks (Birchwood et al 1989; Herz and Melville 1980; Tarrier et al 1998). This is probably because the patients were already in contact with treatment services, hence early detection of prodromal changes could occur. Medication also plays a possible mediating effect.

Data from the Bonn group's longitudinal studies of schizophrenia, which retrospectively assessed onset of basic symptoms prior to the development of definitive schizophrenia, have suggested that onset of prodromal basic symptoms occurs on average 3.3 years before onset of the first psychotic episode (Gross and

Huber 1996; Huber et al 1980). A more recent prospective study from this group found a mean duration of 5.6 years for basic symptoms prior to a threshold diagnosis of schizophrenia (Klosterkötter et al 2001).

It is important to note that the basic symptom theorists state that basic symptoms can also occur independently of onset of full-blown positive symptoms of psychosis, as 'self-limiting spontaneously resolving outpost syndromes', which may or may not be followed some time later by the onset of full threshold schizophrenia. This is consistent with the previous discussion emphasizing that the prodrome is a retrospective concept and that onset of frank psychosis cannot be predicted with 100% accuracy from any particular symptoms or combination of symptoms. Huber and colleagues state that the onset of 'outpost syndromes' occurs on average 10 years before the onset of schizophrenia (Huber et al 1980). Figure 3.2 describes the sequence of events surrounding the onset of psychosis, as described by the Bonn group.

Characterization of the prodrome—summary

To summarize, initial psychotic prodromes are characterized by a wide range of symptoms and great variability between patients. The duration of the prodrome also varies considerably between patients, with some individuals describing no prodromal phase at all, to others reporting a prodrome of up to 20 years. The usual sequence of events leading up to onset of psychotic disorder seems to be first non-specific symptoms, followed by attenuated or subthreshold psychotic symptoms, and finally full-blown psychotic symptoms. Having identified which symptoms are most commonly found and the most common pattern of psychotic prodromes, the next challenge is to identify psychotic prodromes

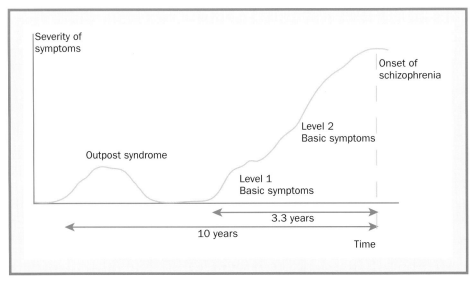

Figure 3.2
Possible relationship of basic symptoms to schizophrenia onset according to the Bonn group.

prospectively, thus enabling intervention and research into this important phase. The important conceptual and practical issues around this task are outlined in the next section.

Recognizing the 'prodrome' prospectively

The 'prodrome' as a risk factor for psychosis

Introducing the term 'at risk mental state' (ARMS)

As was emphasized previously, the term 'prodrome' can only be used once the full-blown syndrome, be it psychosis, hepatitis or whatever, has developed. Therefore, when we shift our focus to recognizing the 'prodrome' prospectively (ie trying to detect incipient psychosis), we cannot use the term 'prodrome'. The term 'prodrome' implies inevitable progression to full-blown illness, and it is clear that no particular constellation of symptoms and signs is invariably followed by frank psychosis. Parenthetically, if such a precursor syndrome were found, it would in fact be best conceptualized as the earliest non-psychotic manifestation of the disorder, and any intervention applied during that period would be seen as early intervention rather than indicated prevention. This issue is more than just semantics. The danger of labelling a syndrome prospectively as a schizophrenia 'prodrome' (or of labelling an individual cross-sectionally as a 'prodromal') tends to reify the syndrome as a disorder or disease, with its own natural history and prognosis (eventual transition to frank psychosis). Instead, the syndrome, which seems like, or could be, a prodrome should be thought of, not as a disease entity, but as a state risk factor for full-blown psychosis. That is, the presence of

the syndrome implies that the affected person is at that time more likely to develop psychosis in the near future than someone without the syndrome. However, if the symptoms resolve then that degree of increased risk remits as well. In an attempt to deal with these issues we have coined a new term, the 'at risk mental state' (Yung et al 1996). This terminology highlights the risk factor approach, suggesting that the syndrome is a risk factor for onset of full-blown psychosis in the near future. The term 'near future' needs clarification too. For how long does the presence of an at risk mental state confer heightened risk on an individual? And how long after it has resolved should the individual considered be at increased risk? Does the individual return to having no increased risk immediately after its resolution or does the fact that an at risk mental state was there mean that the person is at risk for some brief time period after that (1 month? 6 months? 1 year?). The answers to these questions are not yet known, but are currently being investigated in research studies around the world (McGlashan et al 2003; Morrison et al 2002). Our approach to examining these issues will be discussed in the following chapters. Figures 3.3 and 3.4 illustrate the unclear outcome of a cross-sectional at risk mental state and importance of avoiding the term 'prodrome' as a disease-like entity in itself.

Minimizing false positives—the use of enriched samples

It is clear from the retrospective studies of the schizophrenia prodrome reviewed previously that its earliest manifestations are non-specific, for example, reduced concentration, depressed mood, anxiety and so on. These symptoms are found at high levels in the general population

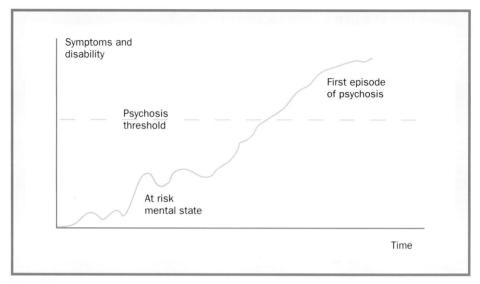

Figure 3.3
An at risk mental state may develop into a first psychotic episode (true positive).

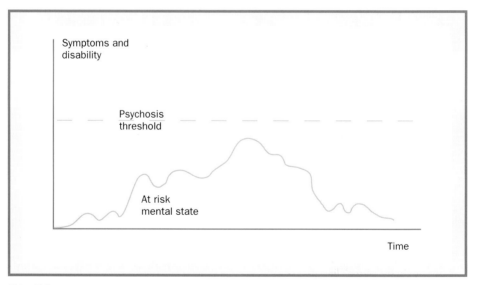

Figure 3.4
An at risk mental state may resolve without developing into a first psychotic episode (false positive).

(Eaton et al 1989; Kessler et al 2001a, b; Meadows et al 2000; Regier and Narrow 2002; Sawyer et al 1990; Weissman et al 1988), as well as in individuals with non-psychotic psychiatric disorders. Hence, at risk mental states with these features alone are not useful from a predictive viewpoint as there will be large numbers of false positives: if individuals with just these features are followed up, the transition rate to full-blown psychosis would be low. Hence, non-specific symptoms do not form a suitable target for indicated prevention. This is particularly so given the very low base rate of schizophrenia and other psychoses (McGorry and Singh 1995; Verdoux et al 1997; van Os et al,1999). Instead, what is needed is some way of focusing on individuals with a likely higher incidence rate of psychotic disorder (Yung and Jackson 1999), that is, gaining access somehow to an *enriched sample* with a likely high rate of transition to frank psychotic disorder.

Several different approaches have been used in the past. The traditional approach is to study family members of patients with schizophrenia (Asaad 1989; Erlenmeyer-Kimling et al 1995; Mednick et al 1987). Thus, a group with presumably an increased genetic risk is identified, and additional risk factors, which make the transition to a frank psychotic disorder more likely, can be examined. This is known as the 'high risk' approach. Assessments usually begin when subjects are children, with follow-up continuing over many years with the aim of detecting the development of psychotic disorder at some stage in the person's lifespan. Mednick et al (1987) modified this strategy by focusing on adolescent offspring who were entering the peak age of risk, an approach that made the high risk paradigm more practical. Researchers using this approach acknowledge that the transition rate to

a psychotic disorder is not likely to be large and results may well not be generalisable beyond the genetically defined high risk group (Asarnow 1988).

A study by the Bonn group examined the predictive capacity of the basic symptoms in a cohort of non-psychotic patients attending a tertiary referral psychiatric setting. Presenting diagnoses were mainly mood, anxiety, somatoform and personality disorders. Subjects were followed up on average 8 years after initial assessment, and over this period over 50% of them had developed schizophrenia. Certain basic symptoms—disturbances of receptive speech, blocking of thoughts, visual perceptual disturbances, olfactory, gustatory and other sensory disturbances—were found significantly more often in the group which developed schizophrenia compared to the group that did not, suggesting that these symptoms may be predictors of schizophrenia (Klosterkötter et al 2001). Thus, this study used an enriched sample of tertiary referred patients most of whom had high levels of basic symptoms. The study's authors regarded them as being 'susceptible to schizophrenia' on the basis of their psychopathology.

A conceptually similar strategy is that of Chapman and Chapman and colleagues, who also attempted to identify hypothetically 'psychosis-prone' individuals on the basis of psychopathology (Allen et al 1987; Chapman and Chapman 1980, 1987). An enriched sample of students with high levels of 'psychotic-like' symptoms (attenuated forms of psychotic symptoms) and isolated psychotic symptoms were followed over time. It was hypothesized that individuals with high levels of these features were at increased risk of psychotic disorder or spectrum disorder compared with controls.

Specially designed instruments were used to assess the level of attenuated psychotic symptoms experienced by the college students who were then reassessed 10 to 15 years later. Results to date have indicated that students who scored highly on scales of perceptual abnormalities and emerging magical thinking were more likely to develop a psychotic disorder 10 years later than comparison subjects. This assessment approach has yet to be developed into a practical method of prediction in real-world settings (Chapman et al 1994).

The 'close-in' strategy

Another approach is that proposed by Bell (1992): the 'close-in' strategy. Bell proposed that 'multiple-gate screening' and 'close-in' follow-up of cohorts selected as being at risk of developing a psychosis would minimize false positive rates. Multiple gate screening is a form of sequential screening that involves putting in place a number of different screening measures to concentrate the level of risk in the selected sample (ie creating an enriched sample). In other words, an individual must meet a number of conditions to be included in the high risk sample—rather than just one, as in the traditional studies. Close-in follow-up involves shortening the period of follow-up necessary to observe the transition to psychosis by commencing the follow-up period close to the age of maximum incidence of psychotic disorders. In order to improve the accuracy of identifying the high risk cohort further, Bell also recommended using signs of behavioural difficulties in adolescence as selection criteria, such as the inclusion of clinical features. This also allows the approach to become more clinical; to move away from traditional screening paradigms and to focus on help-seeking troubled young people who are therefore highly 'incipient' and frankly symptomatic.

The 'close-in' strategy of combining risk factors has been the approach of our group. We have focused on individuals in the peak age range of risk of onset of psychotic disorder—adolescents and young adults (Häfner et al 1994). Other potential risk factors must also be met. One of our enriched subsamples consists of those who, in addition to being in the peak age range of risk, must also have attenuated psychotic symptoms *and* be identified as needing help, either by themselves or by others.

Another similar subsample includes those with self-resolving psychotic symptoms who have been identified as needing help. In addition to these quasi-psychotic experiences being found to occur immediately before the onset of frank psychosis in retrospective studies, there is further evidence of them conferring increased risk of psychotic disorder from the findings of Poulton and colleagues (2000). This large prospective study found that individuals who experienced attenuated or isolated psychotic symptoms at age 11 had increased risk of developing schizophreniform disorder by age 26, compared to those without these symptoms.

Our final subsample consists of individuals with either a schizotypal personality disorder (American Psychiatric Association 1994) *or* the presence of a family history of a psychotic disorder in a first degree relative *and* a marked decline in functioning or marked psychiatric symptoms *and* be identified as needing help. These subsamples are described in more detail in Table 3.2. The exact operationalized criteria for each of these ultra high risk (UHR) subsamples are documented in the Comprehensive Assessment of At Risk Mental States (CAARMS), an instrument designed to assess prospectively and in detail symptoms and signs suggestive of a psychotic prodrome (see Appendix). The criterion of help-seeking distinguishes the first two of these samples from individuals in the general population who experience isolated or attenuated psychotic symptoms but who are not distressed by them and who do not seek help (van Os et al 2000). Thus, the risk of false positives is decreased as well as the potentially stigmatizing effect of being identified as 'high risk' for those not actively seeking help.

We have called the samples that we identify using the close-in strategy a UHR group. The term highlights that the group is different from the 'high risk' groups identified in traditional

(genetic) studies such as the New York High Risk study (Erlenmeyer-Kimling et al 1995). It also tries to convey that we consider the UHR individuals to be at high risk of psychotic disorder within a brief time period (12 months), in contrast to the traditional approach that employs a much longer follow-up period. Our studies so far have indicated that individuals who are referred to the PACE Clinic and meet the above UHR criteria have a cumulative incidence rate of psychotic disorder of between 30% and 40% within 12 months (Yung et al 2003, in press).

With any high risk or ultra high risk approach, there will always be individuals who

Table 3.2
Broad criteria for the ultra high risk (UHR) group

Aged between 14 and 29
Referred to a specialized service for help
Meets criteria for one or more of the following 3 groups:

Group 1. Attenuated psychotic symptoms
- Presence of at least one of the following symptoms: ideas of reference, odd beliefs or magical thinking, perceptual disturbance, paranoid ideation, odd thinking and speech, odd behaviour and appearance
- Frequency of symptoms—at least several times a week
- Recency: present within the last year
- Duration: present for at least 1 week and not longer than 5 years

Group 2. Brief Limited Intermittent Psychotic Symptoms (BLIPS)
- Transient psychotic symptoms. Presence of at least one of the following: ideas of reference, magical thinking, perceptual disturbance, paranoid ideation, odd thinking and speech
- Duration of episode of less than 1 week
- Frequency of symptoms—at least several times per week
- Symptoms resolve spontaneously
- Recency: the BLIP must have occurred within the past year

Group 3. Trait and state risk factors
- Schizotypal personality disorder in the identified individual or a first-degree relative with a psychotic disorder
- Significant decrease in mental state or functioning—maintained for at least 1 month and not longer than 5 years
- Recency: The decrease in functioning occurred within the past year

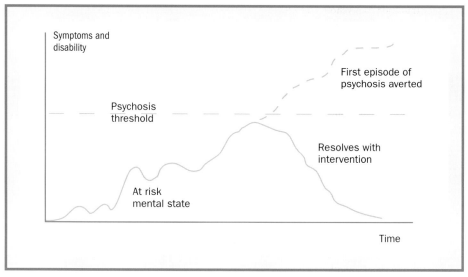

Figure 3.5
An at risk mental state may resolve (eg in response to intervention), but in the absence of intervention would have developed into a first psychotic episode (a false false positive).

Box 3.4
Obstacles to pre-psychotic intervention[1]

- The problem of false positives: there will always be those individuals experiencing an at risk mental state (ARMS) who are not in fact destined to develop a psychotic disorder. These falsely identified individuals may be harmed by being labelled as having an ARMS or as being at ultra high risk of psychosis, and/or receiving treatment at this stage. For example:
- They may become anxious or depressed about the possibility of developing schizophrenia.
- They may be stigmatized by being labelled as 'ultra high risk', by others, themselves or both.
- They may avoid developmentally appropriate challenges (Heinssen et al 2001), for fear of increasing their 'stress' level and risking precipitation of psychosis.
- Similarly, if falsely identified individuals are exposed to drug therapies, especially antipsychotic medications, adverse reactions may occur without benefit.
- If the false positive rate is improved, then the accurate detection rate may conversely decrease. That is, sensitivity may be sacrificed for specificity. This is a mathematical feature of the screening process, even when this is based on encouraging help-seeking for this group. Even with enrichment or successful screening, most of the 'cases' will still emerge from the low risk group.
- We cannot distinguish between false positives and false false positives (in the latter case a true vulnerability exists though it has not yet been fully expressed).

[1] Modified from McGorry PD, Yung AR, Phillips LJ (2003). The 'close-in' or ultra high risk model: A safe and effective strategy for research and clinical intervention in prepsychotic mental disorder. *Schizophr Bull* **29**: 771–790.

make the transition to psychotic disorder, the true positives (about 30–40% on current data), and those who do not, the false positives (see Figures 3.3 and 3.4). We have also described a group called the false false positives (Yung et al 2003: see Figure 3.5). These are people with an at risk mental state who would have developed a psychotic disorder except that some alteration in their circumstances prevented this from occurring. For example, they may have received some form of intervention, stopped using illicit drugs, or had some kind of stress reduction. Thus, they appear phenotypically to be false positives. However, they may have the same trait markers, or markers of liability to psychotic disorder (eg abnormal smooth pursuit eye movements: Lee and Williams 2000) as true positives (Yung and McGorry 1996).

This discussion about false positives highlights that there are potential problems related to pre-psychotic intervention, which are summarized in Box 3.4.

Summary

- The initial psychotic prodrome is often lengthy and is characterized by a wide range of symptoms and variability between individuals.
- Many of the symptoms, particularly in the early prodrome, are very non-specific, such as poor concentration, anxiety and depressed mood.
- Attenuated or subthreshold psychotic symptoms are also found in the psychotic prodrome and tend to occur later, more proximal to the onset of frank psychosis. However, they are also found in a substantial minority of the general population, who may or may not be at risk of a psychotic disorder.

- The initial psychotic prodrome is often a period of marked decline in functioning and potentially health-damaging symptoms and behaviours, such as suicidal thoughts, acts of self-harm, impulsive and aggressive behaviour.
- The prodrome is a retrospective concept— onset of frank psychosis cannot be predicted with 100% accuracy from any particular symptoms or combination of symptoms.
- The term 'at risk mental state' (ARMS) is therefore more appropriate to use for the phase prospectively identified as the possible precursor to full-blown psychosis.
- If ARMS with a high predictive value for subsequent onset of full-threshold psychotic disorder can be recognized prospectively, and effective intervention provided at this stage, then onset of psychotic disorder could be delayed, ameliorated or even prevented.
- However, strategies are needed to increase the accuracy of prediction of psychosis from the presence of an ARMS in order to minimize the false positive rate and the possibility of unnecessary labelling and treatment that this entails.
- Hence, we need to be able to identify enriched samples with relatively high incidence rates of psychotic disorder. One such approach to doing this is the 'close-in' strategy, which uses combinations of risk factors as well as timing investigations to the period of highest risk. In the case of first episode psychosis this is late adolescence to early adulthood.
- Using the 'close-in' strategy we have developed criteria for identifying an ultra high risk (UHR) group, made up of three subsamples. All include help-seeking adolescents or young adults with either attenuated psychotic symptoms, brief self-

resolving psychotic symptoms or a genetic liability to psychotic disorder (schizotypal personality disorder or family history) plus marked psychiatric symptoms or deterioration in function

References

Allen JJ, Chapman LJ, Chapman JP, et al (1987) Prediction of psychoticlike symptoms in hypothetically psychosis-prone college students. *J Abnorm Psychol* **96**:83–88.

American Psychiatric Association (1987) *DSM-III-R: Diagnostic and statistical manual for mental disorders* (3rd edn, rev). Washington DC: American Psychiatric Association.

American Psychiatric Association (1994) *DSM-IV: Diagnostic and statistical manual of mental disorders* (4th edn). Washington DC: American Psychiatric Association.

Andreasen NC Flaum M, Arndt S (1992) The Comprehensive Assessment of Symptoms and History (CASH). An instrument for assessing diagnosis and psychopathology. *Arch Gen Psychiatry* **49**:615–623.

Asaad, G. (1989) Relationship between illusions, hallucinations and delusions. *Integr Psychiatry* **6**:196–198.

Asarnow JR (1988) Children at risk for schizophrenia: Converging lines of evidence. *Schizophr Bull* **14**:613–630.

Beiser M, Erikson D, Fleming JAE, Iacono WG (1993) Establishing the onset of psychotic illness. *Am J Psychiatry* **150**:1349–1354.

Bell RQ (1992) Multiple-risk cohorts and segmenting risk as solutions to the problem of false positives in risk for the major psychoses. *Psychiatry* **55**:370–381.

Birchwood M, Smith J, Macmillan F, et al (1989) Predicting relapse in schizophrenia: The development and implementation of an early signs monitoring system using patients and families as observers: A preliminary investigation. *Psychol Med* **19**:649–656.

Boorse C (1975) On the distinction between disease and illness. *Philos Public Affairs* **5**:49–68.

Bowers M (1965) The onset of psychosis— A diary account. *Psychiatry* **28**:346–358.

Cameron DE (1938) Early schizophrenia. *Am J Psychiatry* **95**:567–578.

Campbell EJM, Scadding JG, Roberts RS (1979) The concept of disease. *Br Med J* **2**:757–762.

Chapman LJ, Chapman JP (1980) Scales for rating psychotic and psychotic-like experiences as continua. *Schizophr Bull* **6**:476–489.

Chapman LJ, Chapman JP (1987) The search for symptoms predictive of schizophrenia. *Schizophr Bull* **13**:497–503.

Chapman LJ, Chapman JP, Kwapil TR et al (1994) Putatively psychosis-prone subjects 10 years later. *J Abnorm Psychol* **103**:171–183.

Docherty J, Van Kammen DP, Siris SG, Marder SR (1978) Stages of onset of schizophrenic psychosis. *Am J Psychiatry* **135**:420–426.

Donlon PT, Blacker KH (1973) Stages of schizophrenic decompensation and reintegration. *J Nerv Ment Dis* **157**:200–209.

Eaton WW, Kramer M, Anthony JC, et al (1989) The incidence of specific DIS/DSM-III mental disorders: data from the NIMH Epidemiologic Catchment Area Program. *Acta Psychiat Scand* **79**:163–178.

Eaton WW, Romanoski A, Anthony JC, Nestadt G (1991) Screening for psychosis in the general population with a self-report interview. *J Nerv Ment Dis* **179**:689–693.

Elias E (1983) Jaundice. In: Weatherall DJ, Ledingham JGG, Warrell DA eds, *Oxford textbook of medicine*. Oxford University Press: 12.175–12.182.

Erlenmeyer-Kimling L, Squires-Wheeler E, Adamo UH, et al (1995) The New York High Risk Project: Psychoses and cluster A personality disorders in offspring of schizophrenic parents at 23 years of follow-up. *Arch Gen Psychiatry* **52**:857–865.

Fulford KW (2001) 'What is (mental) disease?': An open letter to Christopher Boorse. *J Med Ethics* **27**:80–85.

Gross G, Huber G (1996) The true onset of schizophrenia in its meaning for the view of the disorder. *Neurol Psychiatry Brain Res* **4**:93–102.

Häfner H, Riecher-Rössler A, Hambrect M, et al (1992) IRAOS: An instrument for the assessment of onset and early course of schizophrenia. *Schizophr Bull* **6**:209–223.

Häfner H, Maurer K, Loffler W, Riecher-Rossler A (1993) The influence of age and sex on the onset and early course of schizophrenia. *Br J Psychiatry* **162**:80–86.

Häfner H, Maurer W, Loffler B, et al (1994) The epidemiology of early schizophrenia: Influence of age and gender on onset and early course. *Br J Psychiatry* **164**(suppl):29–38.

Hanssen MSS, Bijl RV, Vollebergh W, van Os J. (submitted). Self-reported psychotic experiences in the general population: A valid screening tool for DSM-III-R psychotic disorders?

Heinrichs DW, Carpenter WT (1985) Prospective study of prodromal symptoms in schizophrenic relapse. *Am J Psychiatry* **142**:371–373.

Heinssen R, Perkins DO, Appelbaum PS, Fenton WS (2001) Informed consent in early psychosis research: National Institute of Mental Health Workshop, November 15, 2000. *Schizophr Bull* **27**:571–584.

Herz MI, Melville C (1980) Relapse in schizophrenia. *Am J Psychiatry* **137**:801–805.

Huber G, Gross G, Schuttler R, Linz M (1980) Longitudinal studies of schizophrenic patients. *Schizophr Bull* **6**:592–605.

Kessler RC, Avenevoli S, Merikangas KR (2001a) Mood disorders in children and adolescents: An epidemiologic perspective. *Biol Psychiatry* **49**:1002–1014.

Kessler RC, Keller MB, Wittchen H (2001b) The epidemiology of generalized anxiety disorder. *Psychiatr Clin North Am* **24**:19–39.

Klosterkötter J (1992) The meaning of basic symptoms for the development of schizophrenic psychoses. *Neurol Psychiatry Brain Res* **1**:30–41.

Klosterkötter J, Ebel H, Schultze-Lutter F, Steinmeyer EM (1996) Diagnostic validity of basic symptoms. *Eur Arch Psychiatry Clin Neurosci* **246**:147–154.

Klosterkötter J, Gross G, Wieneke A, et al (1997) Evaluation of the 'Bonn Scale for the Assessment of Basic Symptoms- BSABS' as an instrument for the assessment of schizophrenia proneness: A review of recent findings. *Neurol Psychiatry Brain Res* **5**:137–150.

Klosterkötter J, Hellmich M, Steinmeyer EM, Schultze-Lutter F. (2001) Diagnosing schizophrenia in the initial prodromal phase. *Arch Gen Psychiatry* **58**:158–164.

Kottow MH (2002) The rationale of value-laden medicine. *J Eval Clin Prac;* **8**:77–84.

Lee KH, Williams LM (2000) Eye movement dysfunction as a biological marker of risk for schizophrenia. *Aust NZ J Psychiatry* **34**(suppl):S91–S100.

Loebel AD, Lieberman JA, Alvir JM, et al (1992) Duration of psychosis and outcome in first episode schizophrenia. *Am J Psychiatry* **149**:1183–1188.

McGlashan TH, Zipursky RB, Perkins D, et al (2003) The PRIME North America randomized double-blind clinical trial of olanzapine versus placebo in patients at risk of being prodromally symptomatic for psychosis: I. Study rationale and design. *Schizophr Res* **61**:7–18.

McGorry PD, Singh BS (1995) Schizophrenia: Risk and possibility. In Raphael B, Burrows GD, eds, *Handbook of studies on preventive psychiatry.* Amsterdam: Elsevier: 491–514.

McGorry PD, Copolov DL, Singh BS (1990a) The Royal Park multidiagnostic instrument for psychosis: 1. Rationale and review. *Schizophr Bull* **16**:501–515.

McGorry PD, Singh BS, Copolov DL, et al (1990b) The Royal Park multidiagnostic instrument for psychosis: 2. Development, reliability and validity. *Schizophr Bull* **16**:517–536.

McGorry PD, Edwards J, Mihalopolous C, et al (1996) EPPIC: An evolving system of early detection and optimal management. *Schizophr Bull* **22**:305–326.

McGorry PD, Yung AR, Phillips LJ (2003) The 'close-in' or ultra high risk model: A safe and effective strategy for research and clinical intervention in prepsychotic mental disorder. *Schizophr Bull* **29**: 771–790.

Meadows G, Burgess P, Fossey E, Harvey C (2000) Perceived need for mental health care, findings from the Australian National Survey of Mental Health and Well-being. *Psychol Med* **30**:645–656.

Meares, A. (1959) The diagnosis of prepsychotic schizophrenia. *Lancet* **I**:55–59.

Mednick SA, Parnas J, Schulsinger F (1987) The Copenhagen high-risk project 1962–86. *Schizophr Bull* **13**:485–495.

Møller P, Husby R (2000) The initial prodrome in schizophrenia: Searching for naturalistic core dimensions of experience and behavior. *Schizophr Bull* **26**:217–232.

Morrison AP, Bentall RP, French P, et al (2002) Randomised controlled trial of early detection and cognitive therapy for preventing transition to psychosis in high-risk individuals. Study design and interim analysis of transition rate and psychological risk factors. *Br J Psychiatry* **43**(suppl):s78–s84.

Norman RM, Malla AK (2001) Duration of untreated psychosis: a critical examination of the concept and its importance. *Psychol Med* **31**:381–400.

Perring C (2001) Mental illness. In: Stanford encyclopedia of philosophy. Http://plato.stanford.edu/entries/mental-illness (Last updated 30 November 2001; Accessed 25 September 2002).

Peters E (2001) Are delusions on a continuum? The case of religious and delusional beliefs. In Clarke I, ed, *Psychosis and spirituality: Exploring the new frontier.* London: Whurr: 191–207

Peters ER, Joseph SA, Garrety PA (1999) Measurement of delusional ideation in the normal population: introducing the PDI (Peters et al. Delusions Inventory). *Schizophr Bull* **25**:553–576.

Poulton R, Caspi A, Moffitt TE, et al (2000) Children's self-reported psychotic symptoms and adult schizophreniform disorder: A 15-year longitudinal study. *Arch Gen Psychiatry* **57**:1053–1058.

Regier DA, Narrow WE (2002) Defining clinically significant psychopathology with epidemiologic data. In Helzer JE, Hudziak JJ, eds, *Defining psychopathology in the 21st century: DSM-V and beyond.* Washington DC: American Psychiatric Press: 19–30.

Sawyer MG, Sarris A, Baghurst PA, et al (1990) The prevalence of emotional and behaviour disorders and patterns of service utilisation in children and adolescents. *Aust NZ J Psychiatry* **24**:323–330.

Scadding JG (1990) The semantic problems of psychiatry. *Psychol Med* **20**:243–248.

Subotnik KL, Nuechterlein KH (1988) Prodromal signs and symptoms of schizophrenic relapse. *J Abnorm Psychol* **97**:405–412.

Tarrier N, Yusopoff L, Kinney C, et al (1998) Randomised controlled trial of intensive cognitive behaviour therapy for patients with chronic schizophrenia. *BMJ* **317**:303–307.

Thompson KN, McGorry PD, Harrigan SM (2001) Reduced awareness of illness in first-episode psychosis. *Compr Psychiatry* **42**:498–503.

van Os J, Ravelli A, Bijl, RV (1999) Evidence for a psychosis continuum in the general population. *Schizophr Res* **36**:57.

van Os J, Hanssen M, Bijl RV, Ravelli A (2000) Strauss (1969) revisited: a psychosis continuum in the general population? *Schizophr Res* **45**:11–20.

van Os J, Hanssen M, Bijl RV, Vollebergh W (2001) Prevalence of psychotic disorder and community level of psychotic symptoms: an urban-rural comparison. *Arch Gen Psychiatry* **58**:663–668.

Varsamis MB, Adamson JD (1971) Early schizophrenia. *Can Psychiatry* **16**:487–497.

Verdoux H, Geddes JR, Takei, N, et al. (1997) Obstetric complications and age at onset in schizophrenia: an international collaborative meta-analysis of individual patient data. *Am J Psychiatry* **154**:1220–1227.

Weissman, MM, Leaf PJ, Bruce ML, Florio L (1988) The epidemiology of dysthymia in five communities: Rates, risks, comorbidity, and treatment. *Am J Psychiatry* **145**:815–819.

Yung, AP, Athan E, Graves S (2001) Fever and rash. In Yung AP, McDonald MI, Spelman DW et al, eds. *Infectious diseases: A clinical approach.* Mt Waverly, Victoria, Australia: Cherry Print: 119–128.

Yung AR, Jackson HJ (1999) The onset of psychotic disorder: Clinical and research aspects. In McGorry PD, Jackson HJ, eds. *The recognition and management of early psychosis: A preventive approach.* Cambridge University Press: 27–50.

Yung AR, McGorry PD (1996) The prodromal phase of first-episode psychosis: Past and current conceptualizations. *Schizophr Bull* **22**:353–370.

Yung AR, McGorry PD (1997) Is pre-psychotic intervention realistic in schizophrenia and related disorders? *Aust NZ J Psychiatry* **31**:799–805.

Yung AR, McGorry PD, McFarlane CA, et al (1996) Monitoring and care of young people at incipient risk of psychosis. *Schizophr Bull* **22**:283–303.

Yung AR, Phillips LJ, Yuen, HP, et al (2003) Psychosis prediction: 12 month follow-up of a high risk ('prodromal') group. *Schizophr Res* **60**:21–32.

Yung AR, Phillips LJ, Yuen HP, McGorry PD (in press) Risk factors for psychosis: Psychopathology and clinical features. *Schizophr Res.*

Establishing a service for ultra high risk individuals

4

Having developed draft criteria to identify individuals at high risk of developing a psychotic disorder in the near future, that is 'putatively prodromal', further steps need to be taken in order to provide them with effective treatment. These are:

• Establishing the clinical infrastructure.
• Detecting the target group and promoting service access.
• Engaging the young people with the service.
• Developing and delivering interventions.
• Discharge planning.

Although these steps have been sequentially ordered, they do not necessarily follow one another in this exact manner. In reality, many steps must occur simultaneously, and the strategy behind each step may need to be flexible and evolving, depending on what is occurring in other parts of the system. For example, there is no point in vigorously recruiting ultra high risk (UHR) individuals if the clinical service cannot accommodate their needs. Similarly, novel interventions may be trialed which may require higher staff levels. Case loads must be managed and so effective discharge planning is required. Thus, each component of the system impacts on the others. However, for the sake of simplicity, this chapter will deal with each of these steps in turn.

These issues will be discussed primarily by reference to the Personal Assessment and Crisis Evaluation (PACE) Clinic. The PACE Clinic was established in Melbourne, Australia in 1994 as the first clinical and research clinic for individuals considered to be incipiently psychotic (or at UHR of developing psychosis) (Yung et al 1995,

1996). It is one arm of a comprehensive early psychosis clinical and research programme affiliated with the Early Psychosis Prevention and Intervention Centre (EPPIC) (McGorry 1993; McGorry et al 1996). It has always been an aim of the PACE Clinic to integrate a clinical service for the UHR group with research into this area, just as the EPPIC programme has sought to provide treatment for young people experiencing a first onset psychotic disorder whilst also providing a base for research. Research at PACE aims to examine the process of onset of psychotic disorders, such as schizophrenia, as well as developing interventions around this phase. Obviously, these two research objectives and developing clinical interventions are intimately linked: if we can understand the onset of psychosis and what factors make the transition from at risk mental state (ARMS) to frank psychotic disorder more or less likely, then this may provide the basis for specific treatments for

the pre-psychotic phase. Box 4.1 summarizes the objectives and principles of UHR clinical research programmes.

The steps involved in establishing and running such a service will now be considered.

Establishing the clinical infrastructure

Setting up the service

The PACE Clinic has always sought to distinguish itself from mainstream mental health services which are primarily funded to focus on providing assistance to those who already have diagnosable levels of disorder. Additionally, mainstream services are often viewed in an extremely negative light, particularly by young people. Thus, the name PACE (Personal Assessment and Crisis Evaluation) is deliberately non-confrontational: it does not conjure up any

Box 4.1
Aims and principles of establishing a pre-psychotic clinical research environment[1]

There are several key, interdependent aims of such clinical research programmes:

- To improve the understanding of the neurobiological and psychosocial processes that occur during the pre-psychotic phase and contribute to the onset of acute and persistent psychosis. Conversely, processes, which protect against progression and promote recovery and resolution of symptoms and impairment, may be clarified.
- To improve the predictive power for identification of individuals at risk for a psychotic disorder (either a psychotic disorder in general or more specifically schizophrenia) to better target treatment interventions.
- To develop and evaluate a range of psychosocial and biological interventions to treat current syndromes and prevent future disorders fully expressing themselves.
- To establish a clinical service which is not only highly accessible but also acceptable to young people at ultra high risk (UHR) of psychosis.
- To educate the community about early signs of mental illness in general, and psychosis in particular.

[1]Modified from McGorry PD, Yung AR, Phillips LJ (2003). The 'close-in' or ultra high risk model: A safe and effective strategy for research and clinical intervention in prepsychotic mental disorder. *Schizophr Bull.*

particular images or associations. Rather, it can be accused of being deliberately non-labelling. PACE has also always been located within non-traditional mental health settings, such as generic youth health or community health settings or more recently within a large metropolitan shopping centre. Where possible, clinicians and researchers also try not to limit themselves to working within the office but try to engage with young people involved with the service in their own environment, for example, at their home or school.

Although PACE seeks to distinguish itself from traditional mental health services, it also benefits from close relationships with such services. Indeed, the idea to establish a service for 'putatively prodromal' individuals grew out of, and was consciously anticipated by, experience at EPPIC. It was observed that many young people referred to EPPIC were not frankly psychotic, but were experiencing attenuated psychotic symptoms or other features suggestive of an at risk mental state (Yung et al 1996). Since the mainstream public adult mental health system, including EPPIC, could not provide a service to such individuals who were deemed not 'seriously mentally ill', that is, not sick enough, they were usually turned away. Unfortunately, in some cases the young people re-presented to EPPIC some weeks or months later acutely psychotic. PACE is able to fill this service vacuum by offering treatment to this patient population.

PACE continues to foster collaborative relationships with EPPIC and other psychiatric services. This is important for two reasons. First, UHR young people may be referred to these services by other agencies, which suspect a diagnosis of a psychotic disorder. As indicated above, these people are unlikely to be offered treatment at a mental health service, but they can be managed at PACE. Therefore, other mental health services are an important referral source for PACE. Second, PACE patients who develop psychotic disorders may need to receive ongoing management at one of these psychiatric services, if a psychotic or other mental disorder develops. Good working relationships with other services enhance the handover process.

Although the PACE Clinic has close links with mainstream mental health services for young people in Melbourne, it should be noted that funding for the Clinic has historically derived primarily from research grants. This remains the case ten years after its foundation. It is hoped that in the future, pre-psychosis intervention will be placed on the health policy agenda and will be considered a target for a greater proportion of government funding. An economic analysis of the costs associated with PACE is currently underway including an analysis of savings associated with pre-psychotic intervention compared to intervening after acute psychosis has developed.

Recruiting and training staff

A service focusing on ultra high risk (UHR) young people can be challenging for clinicians. Patients often present with a myriad of problems, 'at risk' versus 'psychosis' status must be constantly monitored, engaging patients may be difficult and they usually cannot be compelled to attend for treatment under any Mental Health Act, unless there is a serious risk of aggression or self-harm. Additionally, there is usually the challenge of integrating clinical and research work. For these reasons it is desirable to recruit some experienced staff to work in such a clinic. The PACE Clinic is also an excellent place for young clinicians and trainees to gain experience, as patients with a wide range of non-psychotic disorders and mental health problems are managed in the clinic as well as patients who develop psychotic disorders.

It is important that all clinical and research staff be familiar with the UHR criteria. Adequate training, including observing interviews using a specialized psychopathology instrument for assessing subtle attenuated symptoms, such as the Comprehensive Assessment of At Risk Mental States (CAARMS: see Appendix), is essential. More junior staff require support and supervision from senior clinicians, and we have found a weekly meeting of all clinical and research staff to be of value. This allows new referrals and existing patients to be discussed and ensures that all staff who are involved in assessments are comfortable applying the UHR criteria.

Detecting the target group and promoting service access

One obvious requirement in establishing a clinical service for the ultra high risk (UHR) population is ensuring that young people meeting UHR criteria are actually referred to the service for assessment and treatment. A key challenge, therefore, is educating potential referrers about the clinical service and its aims, as well as providing education about psychotic disorders in general and the rationale behind early intervention. Such community education has been a cornerstone of the PACE Clinic. Through continual liaison with potential referrers it is hoped that mental health literacy in general is enhanced, particularly regarding psychotic disorders, and that the PACE Clinic is promoted as a clinical service. This in turn should result in referrals to the service.

The community education function at the PACE Clinic has been performed by specially trained clinicians, the 'community education workers'. These clinicians are from a variety of disciplinary backgrounds, including psychology, social work, occupational therapy and psychiatric nursing. It should be noted that this role was first held at PACE by a health promotion worker with a background in marketing and health promotion but no clinical experience. This was not always successful for the reasons indicated below.

The community education role

At present, two part-time community education workers are responsible for the implementation of the PACE community education strategy. It is important to have knowledgeable and experienced clinicians in this role to be able to present information about PACE competently and to be able to respond appropriately to queries. These clinicians also currently fulfil the triage and assessment roles at PACE—they respond to all phone calls from referrers, and determine whether a face-to-face assessment is appropriate and conduct these assessments. This often means that a referrer has already established a professional relationship with the PACE triage workers by attending an information session prior to making a referral and this can help to facilitate this process.

Targeted interaction with key potential referrers

The community education strategy adopted by PACE has been primarily aimed at health, welfare and education services that are in regular contact with young people. A widespread population-based education campaign has not been conducted by PACE due to concerns about the potential of alarming young people and their families about the 'at risk mental state' (ARMS) and possibility of developing psychosis. (A broad population based mental health literacy campaign aimed at young people has recently been conducted in Melbourne—the Compass Program. Its impact is currently being evaluated.) There are concerns that the risk factors for developing psychosis are not yet known with enough certainty to allow any definite statements of risk to be broadcast and a broad community education campaign would result in a large number of inappropriate referrals to the Clinic. In fact, this has been the experience at PACE. There have been several newspaper articles and segments on television 'current affairs' shows over the past few years that have generated a great deal of general interest. However, following this sort of publicity, numerous referrals have been received which have not met UHR criteria.

Targeting potential referrers rather than the general community means that there has already been some level of screening, as the young people referred to PACE are recognized as needing help, either by themselves or by others. It is recognized that there is a risk with this strategy that some young people who meet PACE entry criteria would not be referred to the Clinic because the intermediary service feels that a referral would be inappropriate. It is hoped that the information presented to referrers is clear enough that such situations are minimized. Of course, there remains the possibility that the young person does not come to the attention of any clinical service at all. However, the strategy employed at PACE also ensures that young people referred to the service are those who are seeking assistance or are considered to be experiencing

difficulties warranting clinical input. Thus, asymptomatic young people with a family history of psychotic disorder and people who are experiencing attenuated psychotic symptoms but are not distressed or disabled by them are not referred.

Some direct referrals are received by the Clinic. In most cases the young person concerned is a friend or relative of an existing or past patient of the service who has concerns about their own mental health. In most cases, an assessment is offered to these young people, rather than referring them somewhere else, in recognition of the step made to seek assistance. If PACE is not the appropriate service, they are assisted in identifying one that is.

The bulk of the community education involves linking in with education, health and welfare services and conducting face-to-face professional development or in-service training. Thus, PACE might link in with a network of general practitioners (GPs) and offer to provide training at one of their meetings. On other occasions, PACE might be one of a number of clinical services providing information to a range of clinicians or representatives of services for young people about mental health or psychosis. At these forums information is provided about the aims of PACE, the need for early intervention in psychosis, how to access the PACE Clinic, an outline of research being conducted and the clinical services associated with PACE.

It is important to recognize that community education is an ongoing process. Workers at services change and there are many competing demands for attention and time. To ensure that PACE remains a referral option that is remembered, potential referrers are regularly updated about developments at the Clinic and outcomes of research. There are regular mailings of brochures and other promotional material such as posters and cards broadly outlining the PACE intake criteria. A newsletter, which is distributed on a regular basis to other services, also serves as a reminder of the service. There is also a website that contains information about the research and clinical aspects of PACE that is reviewed and updated regularly and an educational video that follows a young person's pathway through the referral process to receiving treatment has also been developed and distributed widely. The principles and strategies

for community education are outlined in Boxes 4.2 and 4.3.

Referral sources

Young people are referred to the PACE service from a variety of different sources, as shown in Figure 4.1. As mentioned above, it has been beneficial to have a close association with EPPIC and other mental health services in order to be seen as a referral option for young people with mental health problems subthreshold for actual psychosis. Another service change that has been

Box 4.2
Principles of community education

- A strategic approach is used targeting agencies which are likely to come into contact with help-seeking young people. These potential referrers include GPs, school and university counselling services, and other support agencies working with young people, such as drug and alcohol services (Phillips et al 1999; Yung and Jackson 1999).
- Close working relationships with psychiatric services are also important, as ultra high risk (UHR) young people may be referred to these services by other agencies who suspect a diagnosis of a psychotic disorder.
- It is emphasized to potential referrers that they are not expected to apply the UHR criteria themselves, but they if they suspect that a young person is developing a psychotic disorder or is at risk of developing one, then they are welcome to discuss the case by telephone with the PACE triage service.
- A low threshold for face-to-face assessment of a suspected UHR person is applied. That is, if there is any suspicion of the individual meeting the UHR criteria, an appointment is offered.

Box 4.3
Strategies for community education

- Regular professional development sessions at mental health clinics aimed at informing potential referrers about the intake criteria and treatment options available.
- Training sessions for non-mental health professionals (teachers, drug and alcohol workers, accommodation workers, GPs) aimed at enhancing skills at screening for psychosis and at risk mental state (ARMS).
- Development and distribution of community education materials: brochures, posters.
- Development of comprehensive website containing information about intake criteria and treatment options.
- Production of regular newsletters to ensure that the service remains salient to potential referrers and to inform them of any changes to the service.

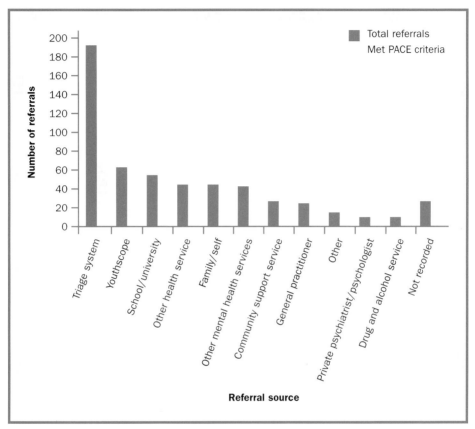

Figure 4.1
Referrals to the PACE Clinic: January 2002–end June 2003.

helpful for PACE is the expansion of the EPPIC service into a youth mental health service, including a clinical service for non-psychotic young people. The whole organization is now called ORYGEN Youth Health, and the 'non-psychotic' arm of the service called 'Youthscope'. Youthscope provides assistance for young people experiencing 'common disorders' (mood and anxiety disorders, substance use problems, eating disorders and so forth) and personality disorders. The development of a service-wide triage system has accompanied these changes, so that a centralized team now screens all referrals to the whole ORYGEN service. This aids the PACE Clinic as referrals can be assessed directly from this triage team, without the need for the young person to be assessed separately by EPPIC or another service managing non-psychotic youth. Referrals can also be made from the various components within the ORYGEN system to its other parts, including PACE. For example, patients are sometimes referred from Youthscope to PACE when it becomes evident that they are experiencing attenuated psychotic symptoms, and occasionally patients are referred to PACE from EPPIC when it is found that they are

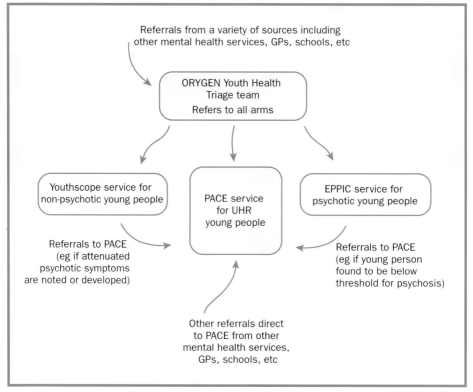

Figure 4.2
Structure of ORYGEN Youth Health and its relationship to PACE.

actually subthreshold for a full-blown psychotic disorder but do have attenuated symptoms consistent with PACE intake criteria. Figure 4.2 shows a diagram of how the different parts of the ORYGEN Youth Health service relate to one another, and the different routes through which entry into the PACE Clinic can occur.

The reader will see from Figure 4.1 that many more referrals are received than actually meet PACE UHR criteria. In fact, no referral source has a rate of greater than 50% of its referrals meeting the intake criteria. This is expected, however, as our approach has been to encourage potential referral sources to refer young people to

PACE when there is any suggestion that they may be at risk of psychosis. The UHR criteria are detailed and difficult to apply if one is not consistently using them. Thus, a low threshold for assessing potential PACE patients is used, and feedback and advice given to the referral source if intake criteria are not met.

Referral process

Initial telephone contact

Potential referrers are always reassured that they are not expected to make the final decision about whether the symptoms experienced by a young person they are concerned about meet UHR criteria or not. In fact, the opposite message is given: the PACE triage team are available via telephone during working hours and are happy to discuss any young people they have concerns about to assist in the decision of whether to formally refer or not. If it is decided that PACE is clearly not the appropriate service, then the triage workers attempt to provide the referrer with information about other options.

The triage workers aim to be overinclusive in accepting referrals for assessment. This is a reflection of the subtle nature of UHR criteria and the recognition that in most cases insufficient information is able to be provided over the telephone to make a valid decision of whether someone meets those criteria or not. This policy has a follow-through effect: the number of young people who are assessed and meet intake criteria is the minority of the total number of assessments performed (Figure 4.3).

Initial assessment interview

Once a young person is referred to PACE and the triage worker feels that a PACE assessment is appropriate, they are then offered a face-to-face interview with one of the PACE clinicians. The aim of this process is to determine whether or not PACE UHR entry criteria are met and to determine the other clinical needs of the young person. Information to assist in this assessment process is obtained from the young person, the referrer, other services as appropriate and the young person's family if possible.

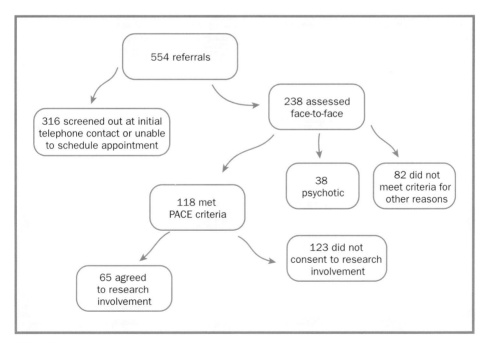

Figure 4.3
Outcome of referrals to PACE: January 2002–end June 2003.

Often, it takes some time to obtain clarity about the young person's current presentation and their history and to determine whether intake criteria are met. PACE clinicians do not feel pressured to make a decision at the first interview if this is not possible. In fact, the full assessment process can take a number of sessions to complete. It is prudent, in some cases, to offer 'serial assessments' to monitor the young person's mental state over a period of weeks or even months prior to involving them in treatment. Young people who are not identified as being at high risk at the time of assessment are also to be encouraged to recontact the clinic in the future if they become concerned—particularly if they have a family history of psychosis or have experienced some psychotic-like symptoms but insufficient to meet ARMS criteria.

Some of the young people who are assessed but do not meet criteria are actually already psychotic and are referred for treatment. Others do not meet PACE criteria but require treatment for another problem and are referred appropriately. Although this process is labour-intensive, it maximizes the number of young people who are accepted into the Clinic. Additionally, it provides an invaluable service for young people and their families in pointing them in the right direction for appropriate treatment if they do not meet PACE criteria.

Engaging the young people with the service

Explaining the rationale for the service

A clinical service for ultra high risk (UHR) or 'pre-psychotic' individuals has a dual focus: (1) treatment of the symptoms and disability that the individual is experiencing currently; and (2) the prevention of full-blown psychotic disorder. These two aspects must be covered when explaining to a young person and their family the rationale for attending the service. Thus, the discussion at the initial appointment at the Clinic must cover the young person's current difficulties and needs and their 'at risk' status. In practice, these two foci are sometimes intertwined. For example, a young person may present with attenuated psychotic symptoms and be concerned not only about their presence but also about whether they will worsen and affect their functioning.

Discussion of presenting complaints

The first component of information-giving and feedback following the assessment process is not usually controversial, and involves discussing a patient's concerns and presenting symptoms, as is the case in any routine psychiatric practice. Often, a label such as 'depression', can help a person feel that his or her symptoms are acknowledged, worthy of treatment and containable, and possibly allow him or her certain exemptions from normal expectations, such as school or work attendance, social gatherings and so on, that is, the temporary adoption of the 'sick role' (Parsons 1950).

Communicating to individuals their ultra high risk (UHR) status

Studies in clinical medicine have shown that people who discover they are at risk of developing a serious illness, such as breast cancer, diabetes, asthma, or Huntington's disease, can develop marked psychological reactions, including anxiety and depression (Jenkins and Conneally 1989; Kash et al 2000; Lerman and Croyle 1994). Thus, in a service for UHR individuals, the potential for such negative consequences of being identified and labelled as at risk must be acknowledged and addressed. The fact that being 'at risk' for a disorder does not mean that a psychotic disorder will invariably follow must be emphasized to patients and their families. Indeed, it is estimated that only between 30% and 40% of patients identified as UHR using the PACE criteria (Table 3.2) will develop a full-blown psychotic illness within 12 months (Yung et al 2003). PACE clinicians tend to tell the young people that they are at higher than average risk of developing a psychotic illness because of certain features they possess (such as family history or attenuated psychotic symptoms), but this does not necessarily mean that such an illness will definitely occur. They are told that there might be other explanations for the symptoms they are experiencing, such as depressive or anxiety disorders, substance use or situational crises. It is important to be aware of the high degree of therapeutic nihilism that remains attached to the diagnosis of schizophrenia. Being able to provide young people and their families with accurate information about psychotic disorders and the high likelihood for recovery with early treatment is a great antidote to this.

The wider implications of their 'at risk' status should also be discussed with patients. Being labelled as high risk for psychotic disorder has the potential to lead to stigmatization of the individual, both by others and by the person him- or herself, a situation known as self-stigmatization. Stigmatization by others if they

learn of the young person's UHR status could lead to problems, such as difficulties obtaining health or life insurance and employment, as well as changes in the way family and friends interact with the individual (Heinssen et al 2001). Self-stigmatization could lead to reduced self-esteem, dysphoria, alterations in life goals, and avoiding the normal challenges of maturation, such as dating, moving away from the parental home, and starting or continuing further education (Corrigan and Watson 2002; Heinssen et al 2001; Warner 2001).

Thus, concerns expressed by some commentators about labelling and stigma (Cornblatt et al 2001; McGlashan 2001) are legitimate and need to be managed by any clinician involved in the 'pre-psychotic' or UHR field. Young people attending the PACE Clinic are assured that their UHR status will be kept confidential and not communicated, for instance, to potential employers or health insurance companies. They are encouraged to involve their families and detailed discussion about their 'at risk' status is held with the family members whom the young person wants informed. Implications of being at UHR of psychosis for various developmental milestones are described and ample opportunities for further discussion with the treating team are provided. This is especially important as degree of risk can alter as symptoms change. For example, if attenuated psychotic symptoms resolve, then the person may be at reduced risk of psychosis, although this is not yet known. The young person's involvement in normal developmental challenges can also be discussed with the treating team.

Case Study 1 describes a typical case and the type of information given at initial assessment.

Case Study 1: Jason

Jason was an 18-year-old apprentice mechanic who had a mother with schizophrenia. He presented to his GP two weeks prior to being seen at PACE because he was having difficulty coping at work and getting on with his colleagues. He had been bullied at the workplace since starting there about five months earlier, and amongst other things had endured his lunch regularly being thrown away, his locker broken into and his personal belongings being vandalized. He became anxious and depressed and rightly believed his workmates were persecuting him. He developed infrequent auditory hallucinations, especially at night, of some of his colleagues' voices taunting him and making derogatory comments. He started to believe that he was 'hopeless' and that even people outside his workplace would think this too. He found himself becoming mistrustful of strangers at times, even though he realized that this was likely to be unfounded and that he was generalizing from his traumatic experiences at work.

His GP referred him to the Early Psychosis Prevention and Intervention Centre, from where he was referred to the PACE Clinic once assessed as not being frankly psychotic.

The PACE Clinic clinician who assessed Jason informed him that he had significant anxiety and depression related to his traumatic experiences at work. He was also told that he presented with certain features which suggested that he might be 'more at risk than the average person' of developing a psychotic disorder, specifically, his family history of schizophrenia and the recent onset of mild psychotic-like experiences. However, he was reassured that he was not psychotic. He was also told that his anxiety and depression would be treated and his unusual experiences monitored regularly for signs of them becoming worse. If this were the case, timely treatment for them would be provided.

Jason welcomed this feedback. He had been concerned that he was 'going crazy like my Mum'. He was pleased to hear that if his attenuated psychotic symptoms got worse that treatment could start at the PACE Clinic and that he would not have to attend the same mental health service as his mother.

Jason was concerned that his 'at risk' status would be communicated to his employers. He was reassured that this would not happen.

Jason brought his girlfriend to his third appointment at the Clinic, as he wanted her to be involved in further discussions about his condition. The couple found it particularly helpful to hear that the symptoms that had been concerning them both (hallucinations and suspiciousness) would be monitored and treated vigorously if they worsened.

In fact, Jason's symptoms resolved once he left work voluntarily. He decided to return to school to complete his final year of secondary education.

Stigma management strategies

Another important factor in engaging young people with a service for UHR individuals is to ensure that the stigma of attending such a service is reduced as far as possible. The information-giving process described above is amongst a number of stigma management strategies which we have implemented at the PACE Clinic. These are summarized in Box 4.4.

Using these strategies, we have found that young people and their families who attend the service do not feel singled out and isolated. In fact, most people attending PACE describe the opposite: they feel that their concerns are being taken seriously and that attending PACE has been a positive experience. This is underlined by the fact that 72% of all young people meeting the UHR criteria attend for three or more visits and 55% agree to involvement in some form of research project (McGorry et al 2003).

Developing interventions and discharge planning

The PACE Clinic offers a case management service which will be described in detail in Chapter 5. Additionally, other interventions for UHR individuals are being trialed both at PACE and at similar clinics around the world, which are discussed in the following chapters.

Summary

- Clinical services for young people at ultra high risk (UHR) of developing a psychotic disorder must be 'youth-friendly', non-stigmatizing and easily accessible.
- Clinical services for young people at UHR of developing a psychotic disorder also need to have close relationships with other mental health services, both as sources of referral of UHR individuals as well as clinical services

Box 4.4
Stigma management strategies

- **Choice of name**: the name of the PACE Clinic was specifically chosen to avoid any direct reference to mental health or psychiatry (Yung et al 1995).
- **Location of the service**: PACE was previously located inside a general medical adolescent health clinic, and is currently within a suburban shopping centre (shopping mall) that is well known and often frequented by young people.
- **Sensitive information giving**: the individual's 'at risk' status is not communicated to them in isolation. It is important to emphasize that psychosis will not invariably occur, that monitoring of mental state is available and that should symptoms worsen timely intervention will be provided as appropriate.
- **Confidentiality of risk status**: assurance needs to be given that an individual's ultra high risk (UHR) status will not be communicated to insurance agencies and employers.
- **Ongoing opportunities for discussion of risk**: it is important that risk status be the subject of ongoing dialogue, as it may alter as symptoms change.
- **Ongoing opportunities for discussion of normal developmental challenges.**
- **Benefits of monitoring and intervention highlighted:** including the treatment of presenting complaints, monitoring of symptoms and UHR status, and early detection of transition to psychosis.
- **Referral networks with other mental health services which also emphasize early intervention and are focused on recovery** (such as EPPIC) to continue treatment of UHR individuals who do develop a psychotic episode.

for these individuals who develop acute psychosis.

- Clinicians working at UHR services need to be well-trained and supervised, in acknowledgement of the varied presentations of the clients.
- Ongoing community education is required to ensure that potential referrers are aware of the UHR clinic. It also assists in educating the community in general about mental health issues. Clinicians should perform this role to ensure that any queries of a clinical nature can be addressed appropriately.
- Community education should be primarily targeted at potential referrers rather than the general public at present.
- The initial screening process should be overinclusive in reflection of the subtle nature of UHR criteria and to ensure that there is minimal exclusion of young people who meet intake criteria.
- The initial assessment should be thorough mental state assessment incorporating information for the young person as well as family and other key contacts if possible. Although the primary aim of the assessment is to determine whether UHR criteria are met, a full clinical picture should be developed identifying all of the needs of the young person.
- Clinicians should not feel that they are required to make a definite decision about whether at risk mental state (ARMS) criteria are met. In fact the assessment process can take several weeks or even months.
- If the young person does not fulfil UHR criteria but warrants clinical attention, they should be provided with assistance in finding the most appropriate clinical service. They

should also be encouraged to recontact the service if concerns arise in the future.

- The young person (and their family if appropriate) should be given feedback about current concerns and symptoms. Information about potential risk of psychosis should be provided in a clear and respectful manner with clients being clearly informed that this is not a definite outcome but a possibility and that there might be other explanations for the symptoms they have described. Wider implications of 'at risk' status should also be discussed if appropriate.
- Steps should be made to minimize the potential for stigmatization of young people and their families who attend UHR clinics.

References

Cornblatt BA, Lencz T, Kane JM (2001) Treatment of the schizophrenia prodrome: Is it presently ethical? *Schizophr Res* **51**:31–38.

Corrigan PW, Watson AC (2002) The paradox of self-stigma and mental illness. *Clin Pyschol–Sci Pr* **9**:35–53.

Heinssen R, Perkins DO, Appelbaum PS, Fenton WS (2001) Informed consent in early psychosis research: National Institute of Mental Health Workshop, November 15, 2000. *Schizophr Bull* **27**:571–584.

Jenkins JB, Conneally PM (1989) The paradigm of Huntington's disease. *Am J Hum Genet* **45**:169–175.

Kash KM, Ortega-Verdejo K, Dabney MK, et al (2000) Psychosocial aspects of cancer genetics: Women at high risk for breast and ovarian cancer. *Semin Surg Oncol* **18**:333–338.

Lerman C, Croyle R (1994) Psychological issues in genetic testing for breast cancer susceptibility. *Arch Int Med* **154**:609–616.

McGlashan TM (2001) Psychosis treatment prior to psychosis onset: Ethical issues. *Schizophr Res* **51**:47–54.

McGorry PD (1993) Early psychosis prevention and intervention centre. *Austral Psychiatry* **1**:32–34.

McGorry PD, Edwards J, Mihalopolous C, et al (1996) EPPIC: An evolving system of early detection and optimal management. *Schizophr Bull* **22**:305–326.

McGorry PD, Yung AR, Phillips LJ (2003) The 'close-in' or ultra high risk model: A safe and effective strategy for research and clinical intervention in prepsychotic mental disorder. *Schizophr Bull* **29**: 771–790.

Parsons T (1950) Illness and the role of the physician. *Am J Orthopsychiatry* **21**:452.

Phillips LJ, Yung AR, Hearn N, et al (1999) Preventive mental health care: Accessing the target population. *Aust NZ J Psychiatry* **33**:912–917.

Warner R (2001) The prevention of schizophrenia: What interventions are safe and effective? *Schizophr Bull* 27:551–562.

Yung AR, Jackson HJ (1999) The onset of psychotic disorder: Clinical and research aspects. In McGorry PD, Jackson HJ, eds, *The recognition and management of early psychosis: A preventive approach*. Cambridge University Press: 27–50.

Yung AR, McGorry PD, McFarlane CA, Patton GC (1995) The PACE Clinic: Development of a clinical service for young people at high risk of psychosis. *Austral Psychiatry* **3**:345–349.

Yung AR, McGorry PD, McFarlane CA, et al (1996) Monitoring and care of young people at incipient risk of psychosis. *Schizophr Bull* **22**:283–303.

Yung AR, Phillips LJ, Yuen HP, et al (2003) Psychosis prediction: 12 month follow-up of a high risk ('prodromal') group. *Schizophr Res* **60**:21–32.

Yung AR, Phillips LJ, Yuen HP, McGorry PD (in press) Risk factors for psychosis: Psychopathology and clinical features. *Schizophr Res*

The clinical needs of ultra high risk patients

5

Although the PACE Clinic in Melbourne has a strong research focus, simply conducting research with young people meeting entry criteria and ignoring clinical needs has never been an option. Not only is this unconscionable from an ethical viewpoint—particularly considering the degree of distress and dysfunction many ultra high risk (UHR) individuals experience—the provision of a clinical service for UHR individuals has been beneficial to the research aims as well.

Ensuring that all young people who fulfil entry criteria for the Clinic are able to access support and treatment for their presenting problems regardless of their interest and involvement in the various research streams has greatly assisted the ability to recruit participants into various studies. Referrers are reassured that the young people they want to refer will not be viewed simply as research subjects but know that their concerns and difficulties will be addressed. This is also thought to be a factor in the ongoing commitment of the young people involved in research at PACE. The fact that, in many cases, mainstream public mental health services have been unable to offer these young people treatment and support because they are not 'sick enough' also enhances their engagement with PACE. The relationships that are established between the young people and their treating clinicians as well as the research team also enhance their commitment to the research component of their involvement at PACE. Often, young people attending the service indicate that they are proud to be involved in research that will not necessarily have a direct impact on themselves, but which will improve treatment for young people in the future.

In recent years, the clinical and research streams of the Clinic have become extremely closely aligned with the introduction of intervention studies that have evaluated the clinical service that is provided.

Clinical resources

The PACE Clinic is staffed by a multidisciplinary team, including psychiatrists, medical officers, clinical psychologists, social workers, occupational therapists and psychiatric nurses. The clinicians undertake a broad range of case management and therapy tasks. This reflects changes within the local mental health scene, in which a case management model of service delivery was adopted about fifteen years ago. Clinical case management in Australia is provided by a range of disciplines including psychologists. Cognitive therapy tends to remain the province of psychologists and, within PACE, psychologists provide both types of intervention. The services of PACE are free, even though the vast bulk of the funding derives from research grants.

In Australia, staffing levels are calculated on the basis of 'effective full time equivalents' (EFT). One full time worker equals 1.0 EFT, a half time worker equals 0.5 EFT and so on. Currently, the PACE Clinic has the following clinical resources: psychiatrists: 1.3 EFT, intake/ triage/ community education workers: 1.5 EFT, case managers: 2.6 EFT. Once accepted at the Clinic all patients are allocated a psychiatrist and a case manager who provide ongoing treatment and monitoring. At the present time there is a standing caseload of approximately 100 young people involved with the Clinic.

The clinical needs of the ultra high risk (UHR) population

Retrospective studies and our own prospective work in the PACE Clinic have found that the symptoms and behaviours that occur in an at risk mental state are extremely diverse and variable (see Chapter 3). In the PACE Clinic studies, young people meeting UHR criteria have been found to meet criteria for a wide range of DSM-IV diagnoses, including depressive, anxiety and substance use disorders, at referral (Leicester et al 2002). Many are also experiencing 'subthreshold' symptoms of non-psychotic disorders, as indicated by moderate to high levels on depression and anxiety rating scales (Yung et al 2003). Table 5.1 shows the range of complaints UHR young people present with upon initial assessment at the PACE Clinic. It should be noted that approximately 22% of PACE clients have more than one DSM diagnosis at initial assessment *in addition to* meeting at risk mental state (ARMS) criteria.

Some UHR patients are able to continue at work or school at some level despite their symptoms. For some this is a struggle, and the young people attending the PACE Clinic sometimes state that they feel pressure to try to continue their regular routine and not to 'give in' to the changes they are experiencing. Others have already begun to decline in functioning and have curtailed or ceased their normal activities. This is consistent with retrospective studies of patients with schizophrenia, which have found that significant psychosocial decline occurs even before the onset of frank psychosis (Agerbo et al 2003; Häfner et al 1995; Yung and McGorry 1996). Recent data from the PACE Clinic illustrates the degree of symptomatology and disability experienced by UHR individuals (Yung et al 2003). A Global Assessment of Functioning (GAF: American Psychiatric Association 1994) of 60.5 indicates a moderately impaired level of functioning, a Brief Psychiatric Rating Scale (BPRS: McGorry et al 1998) score of 19.5, and

Table 5.1
Range of DSM diagnoses ultra high risk (UHR) young people present with upon initial assessment at the PACE clinic

Diagnosis	% of UHR patients[1]
Adjustment disorder	3
Anxiety disorder NOS	3
Binge eating disorder	1
Bipolar disorder II	2
MDE—current	35
MDE—past	15
Dysthymic disorder	16
Generalized anxiety disorder	4
Obsessive-compulsive disorder	9
Panic disorder	9
Social phobia	9
Post-traumatic stress disorder	1
Nil	23

[1]Totals >100 because 20 UHR patients had two or more diagnoses at initial assessment. NOS, not otherwise specified; MDE, major depressive episode.

Schedule of Assessment of Negative Symptoms (SANS: Andreasen 1982) score of 18.3 indicate moderate to marked general psychiatric and negative symptoms, a Quality of Life Scale (QLS: Heinrichs et al 1984) score of 75.8 is consistent with moderate disability.

Compared to first episode patients, PACE UHR patients do not exhibit the same need for crisis assistance and inpatient care. Recent data from EPPIC, which is likely to treat the vast majority of patients presenting with a first episode of psychosis from within the catchment area, show that about 64% of patients managed by EPPIC for a first psychotic episode require an inpatient admission at some stage during the first 18 months of treatment (Edwards et al 2002). This compares with an admission rate of less than 1% in the PACE UHR population.

Case studies 1 and 2 illustrate the different types of presentations and difficulties UHR young people experience.

Case Study 1: Vicki

Vicki was an 18-year-old first year university student who was referred to PACE by the counselling service at her university. She had gone to see the counsellor because she felt that she was not adjusting well to university life and was struggling with her studies. Just prior to commencing university, Vicki had been sexually assaulted by a male acquaintance and this incident was often in her mind. She had not told anyone of this incident until she spoke to the counsellor. She reported feelings of lowered mood, episodes of tearfulness, poor sleep and a lack of enjoyment in most activities. She had withdrawn from one subject because she felt she could not concentrate in class and had not been able to complete a major work requirement. Vicki said that she felt unable to make friends with anyone at university and was reluctant to see any of her old school friends because they were all still friends with the man who had assaulted her. She also said that she preferred to be alone at the present time. Her brother had a history of schizophrenia. Thus Vicki fulfilled criteria for the Family History group but was also diagnosed with a major depressive disorder. Her recent sexual assault was identified as a key issue to be addressed in counselling. She was also treated with an antidepressant medication. After six months her depression had lifted significantly and Vicki was successful in her university studies that semester. She developed a new interest in ceramics through an evening course she enrolled in, and had made some new friends there.

Case Study 2: Ravi

Ravi was a 16-year-old apprentice mechanic who was referred to PACE by his GP. He described increasing levels of suspiciousness and paranoia over the past four months culminating in a two-day episode of intense feelings of being followed by strangers. He said that during that time he had thought that cars going past his house were doing so to keep an eye on him and as a result did not leave the house for that two days. He also described up to three instances per week

of hearing his name called or brief mumbled conversations over the past two weeks. Ravi said that for the past three years he had smoked cannabis every day. His relationship with his girlfriend had ended two months ago after an argument about his cannabis use during which he became violent. Since the break-up of the relationship Ravi reported feeling remorseful and sad and he stated that he wanted to stop smoking. Ravi met criteria for the BLIPS and Attenuated symptoms groups. With the assistance of his PACE psychologist, he identified the following issues for treatment: psychotic symptoms, cannabis use, anger management. He agreed to be involved in the first intervention study at the PACE Clinic and was randomized to the cognitive therapy/risperidone group. At the end of the six month treatment period, Ravi had ceased smoking cannabis and was reunited with his girlfriend. He no longer had the auditory experiences he had described earlier. He continued to experience paranoid thoughts about being followed once a month and recognized that these experiences were more likely when he was feeling anxious.

As the PACE data and case histories illustrate, UHR young people present with a variety of clinical features and syndromes. They are often distressed and disabled by their symptoms. Thus, the treatment provided for UHR individuals should not only focus on the UHR criteria but should aim to address the range of difficulties the patient might present with. Preventing or delaying the onset of acute psychosis in the UHR group might be dependent on addressing both the at risk mental state (ARMS)-related symptoms and other difficulties the patient is experiencing, such as depression. The presentation can also change over time with changing circumstances. Regular mental state monitoring is essential and treatment offered should be flexible to accommodate changes in mental state and functioning.

Clinical interventions in the ultra high risk (UHR) group

Initial assessment phase

As indicated in Chapter 4, following the initial assessment interview a decision is made as to whether the young person meets the UHR criteria or not. This may be done at the time of the interview, or, in cases when there is some doubt about applying the criteria, a decision will be made at a consensus meeting of PACE staff, which occurs weekly. If the young person is accepted into the Clinic, the rationale for attending the service is explained to the patient and family if appropriate. Detailed discussion on this process of information giving and stigma reduction strategies is provided in Chapter 4.

The initial assessment phase also includes assessment of the physical health of the young people. There are many reasons why this is appropriate. First, it is necessary to exclude physical health problems as the basis for their UHR symptoms, particularly before treatment is commenced. Neurological conditions, such as multiple sclerosis and space occupying lesions in the brain, can cause psychosis and psychotic-like symptoms (Lishman 1987). Second, there are

physical health parameters that could potentially be influenced as a result of treatment and this needs to be monitored. Examples are the potential for weight gain (Baptista et al 2002), impaired glucose tolerance (Lieberman et al 2003) and orthostatic hypotension (Wagstaff and Perry 2003) in association with taking antipsychotic medication. There might also be physical health issues, such as pregnancy, that rule out certain treatment options. Thus, all patients need to have a general physical assessment including general physical and neurological examination, and lying and standing blood pressure measurement. A pathology screen including renal, liver and thyroid function, full blood examination and fasting blood glucose is also required. Structural brain imaging (using either computerized tomography or magnetic resonance imaging scanning) is also part of the routine clinical assessment. Thus, the physical assessment of UHR young people referred for help is the same as the routine physical assessment recommended for patients presenting with a first psychotic episode (National Early Psychosis Clinical Guidelines Working Party 2003). Any abnormal results are further assessed and appropriate treatment initiated or referral elsewhere for treatment arranged.

Case management

All UHR patients accepted into the PACE Clinic are linked with a particular clinician or 'case manager' who coordinates their clinical care. The case manager is the day-to-day contact for the young person and provides a link with their psychiatrist, with the research team and with the after hours support that is available. The case manager regularly reviews mental state and assesses risks.

As indicated above, UHR individuals often present with a wide array of problems or difficulties. Often ARMS symptoms are not the young person's primary concern. Instead the main concerns may be relationship difficulties, lack of employment or problems at work, financial stressors, legal problems, problems associated with study, drug and alcohol use, and so forth. The stress associated with these issues might play a role in triggering or prolonging ARMS symptoms and associated psychopathology, including subthreshold psychotic symptoms, and may contribute towards the progression to acute psychosis. Thus, these issues cannot be ignored. Conversely, subthreshold or brief psychotic symptoms could cause or contribute to relationship, employment, education and other difficulties. Indeed, a vicious circle may develop in which both positive attenuated symptoms, such as suspiciousness or other unusual ideas, and/or negative and basic symptoms, such as poor concentration and attention and avolition, may cause social problems. Social problems then result in increased stress levels, which in turn cause worsening of both positive and negative symptoms. Hence, a cascade effect occurs, which could ultimately result in the advent of frank psychosis (Figure 5.1). Thus, it can be seen that a potential target for intervention is to break this kind of cycle, for example, through stress management techniques, which can address the patient's reactions to certain events. Cognitive and behavioural modification could then result in stress reduction and a consequent decrease in attenuated positive and negative symptoms.

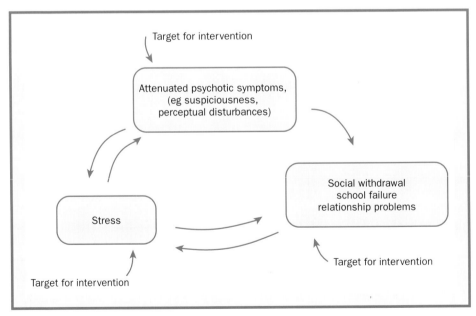

Figure 5.1
The cascade effect of attenuated psychotic symptoms and stress in precipitating a psychotic disorder.

It is not always possible to address all of a young person's problems 'in house' at the PACE Clinic, so the role of the case manager is also to link the young person with external services as appropriate. This can mean that the case manager takes on an advocacy role. Examples include liaising with a school to negotiate a reduced workload and arranging legal advice for forensic- and court-related problems.

Emergency and after hours management

UHR patients are not immune to experiencing crises. Referral to the PACE Clinic often arises during a crisis period—psychotic symptoms sometimes occur in conjunction with a period of extreme distress associated to an event the young person is experiencing. Similarly, crises can arise during a young person's period of treatment with the UHR service or in association with increased intensity or frequency of psychotic features— either a Brief Limited Intermittent Psychotic Symptoms (BLIPS) assessment, or the onset of acute psychosis. In these situations the young person might be experiencing thoughts of suicide or self-harm or may be extremely distressed. Family members can also be distressed and concerned about their relative.

Provisions must be made to deal with these situations if they occur outside regular working hours—for example, during the night or weekends. There needs to be a capacity for support to be offered in these situations via the telephone as well as face-to-face should the need arise. The level of risk associated with the UHR population should not be underestimated simply because the young person might not meet full DSM criteria for a psychotic disorder. This cannot be overstated. It has been the unfortunate experience at PACE that young people attending the Clinic have suicided or made significant suicidal attempts but have not been experiencing psychotic symptoms at the time. This highlights the point made in Chapter 3 about the wide range of symptomatology UHR clients experience—including personality disorder features.

The PACE Clinic is fortunate in being able to draw on the support provided by the Youth Access Team (YAT)—the after hours crisis and assessment team of ORYGEN Youth Health. PACE patients are provided with after hours contact numbers for YAT and are encouraged to call should the need arise. The YAT clinicians assess whether the young person can be successfully dealt with via the telephone— provided with support and counselling—or whether a visit is necessary. In some cases, admission to an inpatient unit might be warranted at these times to contain the situation. The YAT Team are pro-active and responsive. If a clinician has concerns about a client and thinks that some support might be required after hours a referral can be made to YAT to ensure that this happens. They will also respond if the young person contacts them directly. YAT clinicians also liaise with the regular PACE case manager/doctor when appropriate (ie the next day) to ensure that appropriate follow-up can be provided.

Case Study 3 Con
Con was a 15-year-old boy who no longer attended school and was unemployed. He lived with his mother and stepfather, both of whom had schizophrenia. He was

referred to PACE following an overdose of his mother's antipsychotic medication. The initial referral was made to the crisis team in the middle of the night after Con was found by his father shortly after taking the medication. Con was assessed that evening by the crisis team, was assessed medically and support was provided to the family at this time. An appointment was arranged the following morning for Con to meet a PACE clinician the next afternoon.

Con stated that he took the overdose because he was distressed about long-term unemployment, there was a court case pending for charges relating to theft and he had learnt that day that his biological father (with whom he had fallen out) had died. In addition, Con was experiencing mild persecutory ideation (concerned that his family and friends were talking about him behind his back) and infrequent intermittent auditory hallucinations. Thus, Con met UHR criteria for the Family history, Attenuated and BLIPS groups.

Con was linked in with a PACE psychiatrist and a psychologist who also acted as his case manager. In addition to providing Con with counselling and psychotherapy addressing his mood, grief and psychotic-like symptoms, his case manager assisted him in obtaining 'Legal Aid' (free legal advice and representation) for his forthcoming court case. He was also linked in with an employment agency who eventually assisted Con in entering an apprenticeship programme. In addition, the case manager ensured that Con's mental state was reviewed regularly with a particular focus on risk issues. During the early stages of his involvement with the PACE Clinic, Con reacted to increased stress with self-harming behaviours. After hours and weekend support was initiated during these periods whilst he worked with his PACE psychologist to develop better strategies to deal with distress.

Within a short period of time, Con no longer resorted to self-harming behaviours when distressed. His mood and anxiety symptoms also reduced and he became more confident and pleased with the progress he was making as an apprentice and he was able to dismiss any fleeting psychotic-ike symptoms he continued to experience.

Psychoeducation

UHR individuals and their families are usually concerned about changes they have experienced that have brought them to a clinical service. Often, they have many questions about treatment, prognosis and cause. Psychoeducation aims to enhance the understanding the young person and their family have about their symptoms and its potential meaning (Glick et al 1994) and is a core component of UHR services. Chapter 4 provided some details about this. It is important that this information is given in a clear manner so as not to prompt feelings of anxiety or panic. The meaning of being 'at risk', the term 'psychosis' and the possible consequences of being both at risk and developing a psychotic disorder should be discussed. This process needs to be tailored to the existing knowledge base of the individual and the family members and to their capacity to process the information provided. For example, an in depth discussion of possible biological underpinnings of illness can be off-putting and confusing. It can be useful to use an analogy from the physical health domain to illustrate the UHR concept. For example people suffering from asthma have a vulnerability to experiencing episodes of breathing difficulty, which then recede or remit.

Psychoeducation is an ongoing process, adapting to changes in presentation and the phase of treatment. Psychoeducation materials should be reviewed and updated regularly. Information should also always be framed positively—the importance of attending the UHR service should be emphasized and the fact that conversion to acute psychosis is not inevitable should be stressed. Rather, it is important to indicate the dual focus of the service to young people and their families: managing the young person's immediate problems and attempting to prevent progression of symptoms to full-blown psychotic disorder.

Young people often report that discussing their symptoms and possible treatment options in a frank and respectful manner is reassuring and helps them to feel that they have a role in making decisions about their treatment. It can also allay fears and indicate to the young person that they are not alone in the experiences they describe. Such universalization can be comforting (Francey 1999).

Case Study 4: Marco

Marco was a 17-year-old student in his final year at high school. He lived with his parents. His father had a history of major depression with psychotic symptoms. Marco was referred to PACE by his school counsellor because, at times, he had been acting oddly at school. He was generally a competent student who was expected to do well in the final exams at the end of the year. However, his teachers reported that over the past two months, Marco had not completed his work requirements and had appeared distracted at times. When asked about this, Marco disclosed that he had been having the experience of hearing mumbled conversations and on a few occasions had heard a voice talking directly to him making negative comments about his friends and their attitudes towards him. These experiences occurred only up to two times per week for the last three months but Marco was very worried about them because he was aware of his father's history of illness and was concerned that he might also be developing a psychotic disorder. He had not discussed these experiences with his family as he had not wanted to worry them.

Marco was relieved to be referred to the PACE Clinic and welcomed the opportunity to speak about his concerns. He invited his parents to a session with his psychologist and together they were given information about psychosis as well as information about the aims of the Clinic. The concept of early intervention was discussed and Marco and his parents were reassured that his mental state would be closely monitored and if psychosis developed, the appropriate treatment would be commenced without delay. Although Marco and his family remained slightly fearful of this prospect, they were also relieved that treatment options were available for Marco that had not been possible for his father.

Unfortunately, Marco's psychotic symptoms continued to develop despite regular attendance at PACE. He was transferred to EPPIC when his symptoms reached the psychosis threshold and antipsychotic medication was commenced. Within eight months of treatment at EPPIC his symptoms had resolved without the need for an inpatient admission. Importantly, his parents became involved in the family network at EPPIC and were able to support Marco throughout his treatment.

Family work

Family members of UHR young people are often distressed and anxious about the changes they have noticed in their relative. As is the case in managing early psychosis patients, treatment options must therefore have a wider focus than the UHR individual alone. Family work is broader than psychoeducation and might involved addressing systemic-family issues that impact on the young person's mental health.

Where possible, families should be encouraged to be involved in a young person's treatment at UHR services. Obviously, parents are usually concerned about the mental health of their son or daughter and wish to be kept aware of their child's progress and treatment. This should be facilitated as much as possible with respect given to the young person's confidentiality and privacy.

Family members often benefit from being able to speak about the impact the UHR individual's mental health and subsequent involvement with treatment services has had on other family members. Individual family members react in different ways but stress responses including anxiety, depression and grief reactions are not uncommon, much as they are seen with families of first episode psychosis patients (Gleeson et al 1999). Involvement with a mental health service can be associated with great upheaval and uncertainty. Family members should be given time and space to articulate their concerns and feelings if they wish.

Additionally, family difficulties are often identified as a source of distress to the young person and might be considered to be a precipitating factor in the development of ARMS symptoms. Support should be provided to families to address these problems. This might occur in house or could involve referral to a more specialized family service.

Case Study 5: Kylie

Kylie was a 15-year-old girl who lived with her mother, stepfather, and her 20-year-old sister. Kylie stopped attending school three months prior to referral to PACE. She was finding the work more and more difficult and was teased by other students about her poor achievement. She had been unsuccessful in gaining employment and was spending most of her time at home during the day. She reported hearing voices approximately two times a week for half an hour each time telling her to harm herself. She had cut her arms in response to the voices on one occasion. Her mother took her to the family GP when she became aware of these cuts and a referral was made to the PACE Clinic. Kylie met criteria for the Attenuated symptom group.

Over the course of the assessment at PACE, it became apparent that Kylie and her stepfather did not get along well. Kylie's sister spoke of wanting to move from the family home because of the frequent loud arguments between Kylie and her stepfather. Kylie had run away from home on two occasions following one of these arguments, and this was a source of considerable stress for Kylie's mother who had recently been prescribed antidepressants by her GP.

Kylie's case manager (a psychologist) held four family sessions to address the issues that had come to light during the assessment process. An independent service was found for Kylie's mother and stepfather to attend to discuss specific issues related to their marriage.

The psychologist also assisted Kylie in identifying a school that she could attend that was able to offer her increased assistance with her school work. She felt more comfortable in this environment and began to form friendships with other students. As she began feeling happier at home and at school, Kylie reported that the voices stopped occurring and she no longer resorted to cutting herself. She and her stepfather discovered a mutual interest in running and they began participating in local 'fun runs' together.

Parent information sessions held at PACE have also been constructive. Parents of UHR individuals meet together for informal psychoeducation sessions that are facilitated by PACE clinicians addressing psychosis, early intervention and the rationale behind the PACE Clinic and the research component. Adolescence, parenting issues and stress management for parents are also addressed. Different issues tend to arise during discussions depending on the age of the young person attending PACE. For this reason, separate groups are held depending for parents of younger children (aged 14 to 17) from those of older PACE patients (aged 18 or more). Parents are encouraged to speak freely about their concerns and experiences and they are encouraged to ask questions of the clinicians. One of the most beneficial aspects of these meetings is the opportunity for parents to meet each other and to understand that there are other young people who are experiencing difficulties, and other families who are learning to cope with them. Sibling groups are planned for the near future.

Psychological treatment

Evidence is mounting to suggest that psychological interventions during the acute and recovery phase of psychotic illnesses are effective in enhancing the response to drug treatment and the development of adaptive coping strategies (eg, Beck, 1952; Birchwod and Chadwick 1997;

Drury et al 1996; Hodel et al 1998; Hogarty et al 1991; Kingdon et al 1994; Kuipers et al 1997; Lewis et al 2001; Sensky et al 2000). Thus, psychological treatments might be equally applicable during the pre-psychotic phase. Further, psychological treatments aimed at stress management and enhancing coping might be central to the prevention of psychosis in line with the stress-vulnerability model (Zubin and Spring 1977) of psychosis: more details are given later.

Psychological treatment has been a cornerstone of the treatment provided at PACE since its inception. In the intervention trials that have been conducted at PACE, the impact of supportive psychotherapy has been compared with cognitively oriented psychotherapy. Both approaches have their virtues: both focus on engagement and on the formation of a strong, collaborative and respectful relationship between the therapist and the patient and both aim towards the development of effective coping skills.

Supportive therapy

Although it does not specifically target psychotic symptoms, supportive therapy endeavours to provide the patient with emotional and social support and incorporates many of the constituents of Rogerian Person Centred Therapy (Ivey 1988; Rogers et al 1967) including empathy, unconditional positive regard and patient-initiated process. The therapist aims to facilitate an environment where the young person is accepted and cared for and they can discuss concerns and problems as well as share experiences and feelings with the therapist.

In addition to promoting change through non-directive strategies (Ivey 1988; Rogers et al 1967), basic problem-solving approaches are also offered. This may include assisting the patient to develop skills, such as brainstorming responses to situations, role-playing possible solutions, goal setting, time management and so forth (Egan 1994). The patient is encouraged to be pro-active and to monitor his or her own progress. Some degree of role-playing may occur within sessions as a springboard to changes in behaviour outside the sessions. Other examples of problem-solving strategies can be found in Egan 1994.

Supportive therapy with UHR individuals has been shown to be associated with an improvement in a range of measures of psychopathology and functioning after six months (McGorry et al 2002).

Case Study 6: Frank

Frank was a 24-year-old self-employed graphic artist. He lived with his parents and his older brother who had schizophrenia. He was referred to PACE for assessment and treatment by his GP. Frank had been to see his GP because he was aware of changes in his thoughts and emotions in recent times and was concerned that he was developing a psychotic disorder. He described becoming increasingly anxious about financial issues because work had not been as steady as he had hoped. He was planning to marry his girlfriend in a year's time and was trying to save money for a deposit on a house. During the month prior to speaking with his GP, Frank had heard his name called on a few occasions when nobody was around. He had also heard snatches of conversations lasting for around a minute on four occasions over a fortnight.

Frank's therapist encouraged him to speak about his fears and concerns about his career and his concerns that he would not be able to contribute satisfactorily financially when he was married. Frank's fiancée was involved in some of this discussion. Frank and the therapist brainstormed ways for Frank to advertise his business in an attempt to obtain more work. They also discussed stress management skills.

Over time, Frank's anxiety and depressive symptoms improved. Both he and his fiancée reported that their relationship was stronger after they had discussed the concerns that Frank had. Frank also felt that he could share his fears and concerns with his fiancée and not worry about how she might perceive him as a result.

As Frank felt more confident in dealing with situations that arose he ceased experiencing the psychotic-like symptoms. He also was better able to monitor his own stress levels and to assess when he needed to take a break or speak to someone about his concerns.

Cognitive intervention

The underlying principles of cognitively oriented psychological treatment for UHR individuals are to strengthen the individual's coping resources and thus reduce their vulnerability to developing further, or more severe, symptoms, as well as enhancing the individual's understanding of the symptoms they have experienced. There are also broader effects of cognitive therapy on interpersonal and role functioning and self-esteem. The techniques and theoretical underpinnings of the treatment are not exclusive to this therapy, but their integration and application to the UHR population are unique.

The cognitively oriented psychotherapy developed at the PACE Clinic was designed to be provided on an individual basis but could potentially be adapted to suit a group treatment situation. It is conducted over a 6–12 month period, with the frequency of sessions depending on arrangements made between individual patients and therapists, as well as on the mental state of the individual patient.

The stress-vulnerability model of psychosis is central to the treatment (Zubin and Spring 1997). Not only does such a model acknowledge biological factors underpinning the development of these disorders, it also recognizes the role of psychological and social factors. An underlying assumption of the stress-vulnerability model is that ambient/environmental stressors (such as relationship issues, substance use, lifestyle factors) are key factors in the development of psychosis. Moreover, such a model implies that the implementation of appropriate coping strategies may ameliorate the impact of vulnerability factors (Boeker et al 1989). As a result, strategies addressing the experience of stressors and the individual's response are a core component of the cognitive therapy offered at PACE.

Although stress management forms the backbone of this therapy, specific symptoms experienced by patients are also targeted. As the symptoms reported by UHR young people

Box 5.1
Cognitive therapy modules

- **Stress management:** aimed at assisting the client to recognize and monitor their own stress levels, to develop an understanding of precipitants to distress, to recognize associated physiological and behavioural correlates of stress, and to develop appropriate strategies for coping with stressful events.
- **Depression/negative symptoms:** aim at reducing negative/depressive symptoms primarily through cognitive strategies
- **Positive symptoms:** aimed at enhancing strategies for coping with positive symptoms when they occur, recognizing early warning signs of these symptoms, and preventing their exacerbation through the implementation of preventive strategies.
- **Other comorbidity:** addresses other problem areas commonly experienced by UHR clients, such as social anxiety, generalized anxiety, panic disorder (or symptoms of panic attacks), obsessive-compulsive symptoms, post-traumatic symptoms, and substance use.

vary widely, therapists working with this population need to be able to 'customize' the psychological treatment that is offered. For this reason, a number of treatment modules have been developed within the cognitive therapy: *Stress management, Depression/negative symptoms, Positive symptoms* and *Other comorbidity*. The selection of modules to be implemented during the course of therapy with an individual is informed by an assessment of the presenting problem(s) and the patients' own perception of their functioning. The cognitive therapy is presented in more detail elsewhere (Phillips and Francey in press) and in Box 5.1.

Cognitive oriented therapy, in conjunction with antipsychotic treatment, has been associated with a significantly lower rate of transition to acute psychosis compared to the supportive therapy described above (McGorry et al 2002). This effect was held only whilst the two treatments were actually being offered—6 months after treatment was withdrawn, the difference diminished. Fifty-five per cent of the cognitive therapy plus risperidone group were either only partially compliant with the antipsychotic or totally non-compliant. It can therefore be inferred that cognitive therapy had an impact on the symptoms and functioning of this group—at least while it was offered. A study comparing cognitive therapy alone with supportive therapy is currently underway at PACE. Meanwhile, in Manchester, UK the Early Detection and Intervention Evaluation (EDIE) group have compared the impact of cognitive-behaviour oriented psychotherapy with monitoring alone (ie, no psychological treatment) on the rate of transition to psychosis in 23 young people meeting ARMS criteria (French 2002; Morrison et al 2002). After 26 sessions of cognitive-behavioural therapy only one of the 13 participants (8%) in this group had developed acute psychosis. This compared to four of the 11 in the monitoring group (36%) (French 2002).

To date, cognitive therapy at PACE has only been offered on an individual basis. Group psychotherapy might be useful to address social anxiety, social skills training and some aspects of stress management.

Case Study 7: Jana

Jana was a 23-year-old shop assistant who reported that she occasionally believed that she could foresee the future. For example, she thought that she could influence the songs that were played on the radio and that by thinking about a friend, that friend would call her on the telephone. These beliefs had arisen over the past year but had not been present continuously over that time. Most of the time she was able to question the likelihood of influencing the behaviour of others but she reported one occasion lasting for two days when she was overwhelmed by what she believed were examples of her ability to control what was happening around her. This feeling of being overwhelmed resulted in her being unable to attend work for the two day period. She was later able to recognize that her beliefs were unfounded.

Jana and her therapist devised a test of her 'powers'. During a series of sessions they listened to a radio station and Jana predicted what songs were going to be played. Her accuracy rate was less than 5%. This convinced her that she could not influence the radio station. Jana and her therapist also tested her 'ability' to subconsciously encourage her friends to call her. They worked out a timetable of times when Jana was to think about a particular friend. She was to record whether that friend telephoned her at this time. There were very few examples of a friend calling after Jana had thought about them. Both of these tasks led Jana

to question that what she had believed were special powers did not exist.

Psychopharmacological treatment

To date, the only published clinical trials conducted in the UHR population have used antipsychotic medication. The first, by McGorry and colleagues at PACE (McGorry et al 2002) was a randomized controlled trial (RCT) of combined intensive cognitive therapy plus low dose risperidone, compared to a 'treatment as usual' (supportive case management) arm. At the end of the 6 month treatment phase, significantly more subjects in the 'treatment as usual' group had developed an acute psychosis than in the intervention group (p = .026). This difference was no longer significant at the end of a post treatment 6 month follow-up period (p = .16), although it did remain significant for the risperidone-adherent subgroup of cases. This result suggests that it is possible to delay the onset of acute psychosis with intervention. Both groups experienced a decrease in symptoms and improved functioning over the treatment and follow-up phases, compared to entry levels. There is currently a further intervention trial underway at PACE which is attempting to distil the active ingredient from the first study by separating the psychological and pharmacological treatment components.

A double blind RCT of olanzapine in a 'prodromal' group has recently been completed by the Prevention Through Risk Identification Management and Education (PRIME) team (McGlashan et al 2003; Miller et al 2003; Woods et al in press). Preliminary results of this trial indicate that UHR patients benefit from the provision of antipsychotic medication—in this case olanzapine (Woods et al 2002, in press). Twenty UHR patients who received olanzapine reported lower levels of 'prodromal' symptomatology after 8 weeks of treatment than 21 UHR patients who received placebo medication. Further results from this study are anticipated.

Although antipsychotic medication is an obvious choice due to its efficacy in treating established psychotic disorders and particularly threshold positive symptoms, other interventions may be more appropriate for early stages of illness (Berger et al 2002; Kane et al in press; McGorry et al 2001). Indeed, frank psychotic symptoms may just be 'noise' around an underlying disease process that could respond to something quite different from antipsychotic medication. Use of antipsychotics in the high risk group, even in those truly experiencing emerging psychosis may be analogous to treating a person's angina pectoris with glyceryl trinitrate (GTN). Generally, the patient feels better, but the underlying disease process (ischaemic heart disease) is not treated and continues unabated, leaving the person at risk of relapse (Yung 2003). Indeed, the next episode may be more severe and less amenable to treatment, since the underlying disease has progressed, again a situation we often see in schizophrenia (Lieberman, 1999).

Thus, alternatives to antipsychotic medication also need to be considered as possible treatment options for the UHR population. Investigators at the Hillside-Recognition and Prevention (Hillside-RAP) Clinic in New York believe that the development of specific preventive interventions is premature at present. Instead, they have chosen a 'naturalistic'

approach to studying the appropriateness and efficacy of various potential treatments for UHR young people. Thus, they have surveyed the treatment provided to young people meeting RAP criteria by psychiatrists but have not sought to direct the type of treatment provided. The mental state of over 80% of the patients recruited to RAP has either improved or stabilized over time (Cornblatt et al 2002). Over 80% of patients received a pharmacological treatment, either antipsychotic medication or antidepressants, with both demonstrating clinical improvement (Cornblatt et al 2002). The authors of this study suggest that this indicates that antidepressants may be effective in treating the underlying vulnerability of schizophrenia and should be considered when developing preventive interventions. It should be noted that many of these young people—particularly the group labelled as 'schizophrenia-like psychosis' or SLP—would be viewed as already psychotic within the PACE framework.

Additionally, neuroprotective agents may be of benefit in the UHR group. The theory behind such an approach is that dysfunctional regulation of generation and degeneration in some brain areas might explain neurodevelopmental abnormalities seen in early psychosis (Berger et al in press). (Further information about this model is provided in Chapter 6.) Neuroprotective strategies countering the loss or supporting the generation of progenitor cells may therefore be a potent therapeutic avenue to explore. Substances that regulate the generation and death of cells, such as lithium (Manji et al 1999), eicosapentanoic acid (EPA: Fenton et al 2000), and glycine (Javitt et al 2001) might therefore have a role in preventing the onset of illness in the UHR population. Open labelled studies using lithium and EPA are now underway in

Melbourne and Yale (Woods, pers comm, Colorado Springs, 2003), respectively, in the first steps towards evaluating the efficacy of these substances in both preventing the onset of psychosis in UHR cohorts and in improving mental state.

Other treatment options have yet to be tested in the UHR population. Consistent with the stress-diathesis model of schizophrenia (Nicholson and Neufeld 1992; Nuechterlein and Dawson 1984; Zubin and Spring 1977) other candidate treatments include corticotrophin-releasing hormone (CRH) receptor agonists (Corcoran et al in press). Furthermore, a recent study has suggested that oestrogen may be effective as an adjunctive treatment to atypical antipsychotic medications in reducing the psychotic symptoms experienced by women with established psychosis (Kulkarni et al 2001, 2002). Oestrogen might therefore have a role in the treatment of UHR women.

Treatment of presenting symptoms

As indicated above, UHR individuals present to the PACE Clinic with a variety of symptoms and syndromes. Depression is a common feature. Management of current problems is a core function of the Clinic, in addition to the aim of psychosis prevention, amelioration or delay. Non-pharmacological approaches have already been described. In addition, UHR patients do sometimes need treatment with medication such as antidepressants and anti-anxiety agents. Antipsychotic medication is presently used only in the context of a clinical trial, where informed consent to the research goal is explicitly required. The possible exceptions to this are situations when a UHR young person has developed worsening

attenuated psychotic symptoms in addition to severe suicidal or homicidal ideation that may be related to the content of symptomatology (see the draft clinical guidelines below). Indeed, this is the approach of the PRIME Clinic, where patients are in fact deemed to be 'psychotic', or to have 'converted', if they develop marked suicidality and/or dangerousness in conjunction with attenuated psychotic symptoms (Miller et al 2002, in press).

Currently, it is too early for codifying firm guidelines and recommendations regarding psychopharmacological treatment for UHR individuals. Although antipsychotic medications have been demonstrated to have some efficacy with this population, more research is required to determine when this is really necessary and also for how long treatment should be provided. Combinations of medical treatments have yet to be considered. Further, it is possible that different types of medication could have different levels of efficacy in preventing transition to psychosis or in improving mental state in general, depending on the symptom profile of individual patients, duration of symptoms, side-effect profiles and so forth. Firm recommendations for treatment will only be forthcoming after considerably more research. There still may be a need to offer conservative treatment strategies in the interim.

Termination and discharge

As mentioned above, guidelines for the duration of individuals who meet UHR criteria have not yet been determined. Intervention studies that have so far been conducted have provided treatment for 6 or 12 months (McGlashan et al 2003; McGorry et al 2002; Morrison et al 2002).

In practice, termination of treatment is guided by reduction or resolution of symptoms and patient preferences. Over the years it has been seen that patients who attend PACE and who do not develop a psychotic disorder have varying levels of need for continued treatment once their 'episode of care' at the PACE Clinic has ended. In some cases, an individual might be struggling with some of the issues or symptoms that were present when they first attended PACE, such as episodic depression. In other cases although frank psychosis did not develop, another Axis 1 disorder has emerged. In still other cases, personality pathology becomes more prominent and apparent as the period of treatment at PACE continues.

In practice, the presentation of an individual, as well as treatment options that are available, determines the follow-up that is arranged once a decision is made that PACE is no longer the most appropriate service. Some young people will require no further treatment. However, it is common practice at discharge to encourage young people to recontact PACE in the future if they or their family become concerned about their mental state. The rationale for this is that they are assumed to be more likely to contact clinicians and a clinical service they are already familiar with if a crisis develops or symptoms re-emerge. PACE clinicians can then assess the situation and determine what level of treatment is required at this stage. In a number of cases, patients or their families have been in contact post discharge and it has become apparent that the young person is experiencing an acute psychotic episode. If this is the case, the PACE clinician can quickly refer the individual to the appropriate service and thereby minimize delays in treatment.

Case Study 8: May-Ling

May-Ling was an 18-year-old university student who shared a house with friends. She reported experiencing a 48 hour period of intense paranoia following an argument with her boyfriend. She became convinced that her housemates wanted to physically harm her and had hired a hit man to do this. Over this period, she secluded herself in her bedroom staying away from windows as she was convinced that cars passing by were full of assassins. After 48 hours these thoughts subsided and May-Ling was able to recognize that they were unfounded beliefs. She spoke with a counsellor at university who referred her to PACE.

May-Ling was treated at PACE for 12 months. Over this time, she was prescribed a low dose antipsychotic medication (as part of a clinical trial) and received counselling. Her family and boyfriend were invited to a number of sessions with May-Ling.

After 12 months she was discharged from the Clinic. She had returned to her university studies after a short break and was living with a close friend. She continued going out with her boyfriend. There had been no evidence of psychotic symptoms over her treatment period.

Eight months after discharge, however, May-Ling's mother contacted PACE saying that she was extremely concerned abut May-Ling who had recently broken up with her boyfriend. She said that over the past week May-Ling had barely left her house and only did so with someone else. She had not been eating or sleeping well and was not attending to her personal hygiene. An appointment was made for later that day and May-Ling's psychologist and psychiatrist went to her house to see her. It was felt that May-Ling was very unwell. Her persecutory thoughts had returned and May-Ling was extremely fearful of her housemate. She was worried that people who passed by the house were keeping an eye on her with a view to physically harming her if she left the house. Thus, May-Ling was thought to be psychotic at this stage and treatment was immediately arranged for her.

Draft clinical guidelines for treatment

Guidelines for the treatment of young people meeting UHR criteria have been developed (Box 5.2). These guidelines are in their early formative state and should be considered a 'work in progress', which will be refined as experience working with this population develops and becomes more widespread.

Box 5.2
Draft guidelines for treatment and research with young people at ultra high risk (UHR) of developing a psychotic disorder[1]

- Young people who are distressed by signs and symptoms of an at risk mental state (ARMS) and are seeking treatment should be:
  - engaged and assessed by a mental health service that is aware of the unique needs of this clinical group;
  - offered regular monitoring of mental state;
  - offered specific treatment for syndromes, such as depression, anxiety or substance misuse, and assistance with other problem areas as necessary (such as interpersonal, vocational and family-related);
  - provided with psychoeducation and support to better understand the symptoms they have experienced;
  - offered treatment to assist in developing skills to cope with subthreshold psychotic symptoms that might be experienced;
  - offered family education and support
  - provided with information in a flexible, clear and careful way about risks for mental disorders, as well as existing syndromes;
  - provided with appropriate treatment with minimal delay if symptoms worsen and an acute psychotic episode develops.
- Treatment of ultra high-risk (UHR) patients/clients should be carried out in a low stigma environment, such as home, primary care or a youth-friendly office based setting.
- Antipsychotic medication should not generally be considered as the first treatment option for the UHR population at present, in recognition of the need for further evaluation of the appropriateness and efficacy of this treatment. Exceptions are:

Box 5.2
(continued)

> – when there is rapid deterioration of mental state;
> – when severe suicidal risk is present and treatment of depression has proved ineffective;
> – when aggression or hostility are increasing and proving a threat to others.
> • If antipsychotic medication is considered, low dose atypical medication should be used. If there is benefit and resolution of symptoms after 6 weeks, the medication can be continued for between 6 months and 2 years with the patient's consent. After this period, if there has been a good recovery and the patient is agreeable, the medication should be gradually withdrawn. If there has been no or limited response to one atypical antipsychotic medication, this strategy should be carefully reviewed and another can be trialed if the above indications still exist.
> • If young people with an at risk mental state (ARMS) are not seeking or willing to accept help themselves, it might be appropriate to offer support and education to family and friends.
> • The evidence of the efficacy of treatments aimed specifically at reducing the risk of transition to psychosis (antipsychotic medication, cognitive and family therapy or other experimental neuroprotective drug strategies) remains preliminary. More evidence is required and the risk/benefit ratio of various interventions needs to be more accurately determined.
>
> *Research*
> • The process of development of acute psychosis from premorbid and prodromal mental states needs to be better characterized from phenomenological, psychosocial and neurobiological levels.
> • Further research is required to determine which treatment strategies are effective in reducing the burden of symptoms and disability experienced by individuals with an ARMS and in reducing the risk of progression to a psychotic disorder.
> • This research must meet the highest ethical standards applicable to all medical research. Patients must be given genuine informed consent and be free to withdraw from research at any time. Non-participation in research must not affect access to appropriate clinical care. Research should be led by local clinicians and researchers so that culturally normal experiences and behaviours are not misconstrued as signs and symptoms of illness.
>
> [1]Adapted from Edwards J, McGorry PD (2002) *Implementing early intervention in psychosis: A guide to establishing early psychosis services.* Martin Dunitz: London. McGorry PD, Killackey E, Elkins K, Lambert M, Lambert T (2003) Summary Australian and New Zealand clinical practice guidelines for the treatment of schizophrenia. *Austral Psychiatry* 11:136–147.

Summary

• Young people meeting ultra high risk (UHR) criteria should be able to access support and treatment for presenting problems regardless of their interest and involvement in research studies.
• The clinical needs of ultra high risk (UHR) patients are wide-reaching and diverse. Data from the PACE Clinic indicates that UHR individuals experience moderate levels of functioning and disability and moderate to marked levels of psychiatric symptoms.
• Assessment of young people referred to UHR services should include an assessment of their physical health as well as their mental health.
• UHR individuals often have concerns above and beyond their ARMS symptoms, such as legal, housing, drug and alcohol use and so forth, which might play a role in triggering or

prolonging ARMS symptoms and other psychopathology. In some cases, external services might be drawn upon to assist with these issues.

- After hours and emergency support should be available to UHR patients as required.
- Educating the young person and their family about their 'at risk' status and other mental health issues is an important cornerstone of treatment.
- If possible, treatment should not just focus on the young person but also their family network providing assistance and support to other family members as appropriate.
- Psychological treatment—both supportive therapy and cognitive oriented strategies—is important in assisting engagement and addressing presenting symptoms.
- Pharmacology trials with the UHR population suggest that medication might play a role in treatment of this group of young people. However, there are very few studies to date and those that have been reported have been limited to antipsychotic medication. Further work is required in this area before clear guidelines are available for the use of antipsychotics and other drugs outside of clinical trials.
- The need for treatment might extend beyond what is available at a specialist UHR clinical service. Discharge planning and the identification of ongoing support and care needs to commence well before the anticipated discharge date.

References

Agerbo E, Byrne M, Eaton WW, Mortensen PB (2003) Schizophrenia, marital status and employment: A forty year study. *Schizophr Res* **60**(suppl):32.

American Psychiatric Association (1994) *DSM-IV: Diagnostic and Statistical Manual of Mental Disorders* (4th edn). Washington DC: American Psychiatric Association.

Andreasen N (1982) Negative symptoms in schizophrenia: Definition and reality. *Arch Gen Psychiatry;* **39**:784–788.

Baptista T, Kin NM, Beaulieu S, de Baptista EA (2002) Obesity and related metabolic abnormalities during antipsychotic drug administration: mechanisms, management and research perspectives. *Pharmacopsychiatry* **35**:205–219.

Beck AT (1952) Successful outpatient psychotherapy of a chronic schizophrenic with a delusion based on borrowed guilt. *Psychiatry* **15**:305–312.

Berger GE, Wood SJ, Pantelis C, et al (2002) Implications of lipid biology for the pathogenesis of schizophrenia. *Aust NZ J Psychiatry* **36**:355–366.

Berger GE, Wood S, McGorry PD (in press) Incipient neurovulnerability and neuroprotection in early psychosis. *Psychopharmacol Bull*

Birchwood M, Chadwick P (1997) The omnipotence of voices: Testing the validity of a cognitive model. *Psychol Med* **27**:1345–1353.

Boeker W, Brenner HD, Wuergler S (1989) Vulnerability-linked deficiencies, psychopathology and coping behaviour of schizophrenics and their relatives. *Br J Psychiatry* **155**(suppl 5):128–135.

Corcoran C, Walker E, Huot R, et al (in press) The stress cascade and schizophrenia: Etiology and onset. *Schizophr Bull*

Cornblatt B, Lencz T, Correll C, et al (2002) Treating the prodrome: Naturalistic findings from the RAP Program. *Acta Psychiatr Scand Suppl* **106**:44.

Drury V, Birchwood M, Cochrane R, MacMillan F (1996) Cognitive therapy and recovery from acute psychosis: A controlled trial: I. Impact on psychotic symptoms. *Br J Psychiatry* **169**:593–601.

Edwards J, Harris M, Herman A (2002) The Early Psychosis Prevention and Intervention Centre, Melbourne, Australia: An overview, November 2001. In Ogura C, ed, *Recent advances in early intervention and prevention in psychiatric disorders*. Tokyo: Siewa Shoten Publishers: 26–33.

Edwards J, McGorry PD (2002) *Implementing early intervention in psychosis: A guide to establishing early psychosis services.* Martin Dunitz: London.

Egan G (1994) *The skilled helper: A problem-management approach to helping* (5th edn) Pacific Grove, CA: Brooks/Cole.

Fenton WS, Hibbel J, Knable M (2000) Essential fatty acids, lipid membrane abnormalities, and the diagnosis and treatment of schizophrenia. *Biol Psychiatry* 47:8–21.

Francey SM (1999) The role of day programmes in recovery in early psychosis. In McGorry PD, Jackson HJ, eds, *The recognition and management of early psychosis: A preventive approach.* Cambridge University Press: 407–437.

French P (2002) Model-driven psychological intervention to prevent onset of psychosis. *Acta Psychiatr Scand Suppl* 106:18.

Gleeson J, Jackson HJ, Stavely H, Burnett P (1999) Family intervention in early psychosis. In McGorry PD, Jackson HJ, eds, *The recognition and management of early psychosis: A preventive approach.* Cambridge University Press: 376–406.

Glick ID, Burti L, Okonogi K, Sacks M (1994) Effectiveness in psychiatric care: III. Psychoeducation and outcome for patients with major affective disorder and their families. *Br J Psychiatry* 164:104–106.

Häfner H, Nowotny B, Loffler W, et al (1995) When and how does schizophrenia produce social deficits? *Eur Arch Psychiatry Clin Neurosci* 246:17–28.

Heinrichs DW, Hanlon TE, Carpenter WT (1984) The Quality of Life Scale: an instrument for rating the schizophrenic deficit syndrome. *Schizophr Bull* 10:388–398.

Hobbs C, Newton L Tennant C, et al (2002) Deinstitutionalization for long-term mental illness: a 6-year evaluation. *Aust NZ J Psychiatry* 36:30–36.

Hodel B, Brenner HD, Merlo MCG, Teuber JF (1998). Emotional management therapy in early psychosis. *Br J Psychiatry* 172(suppl):128–133.

Hogarty GE, Anderson CM, Reiss DJ, et al (1991) Family psychoeducation, social skills training and maintenance chemotherapy in the aftercare treatment of schizophrenia. *Arch Gen Psychiatry* 48:340–347.

Ivey AE (1988) *Intentional interviewing and counseling.* Pacific Grove, CA: Brooks/Cole.

Javitt DC, Silipo G, Cienfuegos A, et al (2001) Adjunctive high-dose glycine in the treatment of schizophrenia. *Int J Neuropsychopharmacol* 4:385–391.

Kane JM, Krystal J. Schooler N, Correll C (in press) Pharmacologic treatment models and designs. *Schizophr Bull*

Kingdon D, Turkington D, John C (1994) Cognitive behaviour therapy of schizophrenia: The amenability of delusions and hallucinations to reasoning. *Br J Psychiatry* 164:581–587.

Kuipers E, Garety P, Fowler DF, et al (1997) London-East Anglia randomised controlled trial of cognitive-behavioural therapy for psychosis. *Br J Psychiatry* 171:319–327.

Kulkarni J, Riedel A, de Castella AR, et al (2001) Estrogen: A potential treatment for schizophrenia. *Schizophr Res* 48:137–144.

Kulkarni J, Riedel A, de Castella AR, et al (2002) A clinical trial of adjunctive oestrogen treatment in women with schizophrenia. *Arch Women's Mental Health* 5:99–104.

Leicester SB, Amminger GP, Phillips LJ, et al (2002) *DSM-IV Axis I disorders in individuals at ultra-high risk for psychosis.* Paper presented at the 3rd International Early Psychosis Conference, Copenhagen, Denmark, September.

Lewis SW, Tarrier N, Haddock G, et al (2001) A randomised controlled trial of cognitive behavior therapy in early schizophrenia. *Schizophr Res* 49:263.

Lieberman JA (1999) Pathophysiologic mechanisms in the pathogenesis and clinical course of schizophrenia. *J Clin Psychiatry* 60(suppl):9–12.

Lieberman JA, Tollefson G, Tohen M, et al (2003) Comparative efficacy and safety of atypical and conventional antipsychotic drugs in first-episode psychosis: A randomised, double-blind trial of olanzapine versus haloperidol. *Am J Psychiatry* 160:1396–1404.

Lishman WA (1987) *Organic psychiatry: The psychological consequences of cerebral disorder* (2nd edn). Oxford: Blackwell.

Manji HK, Moore GJ, Chen G. (1999) Lithium at 50: Have the neuroprotective effects of this unique medication been overlooked? *Biol Psychiatry* **46**:929–940.

McGlashan TH, Zipursky RB, Perkins D, et al (2003) The PRIME North America randomized double-blind clinical trial of olanzapine versus placebo in patients at risk of being prodromally symptomatic for psychosis: I. Study rationale and design. *Schizophr Res* **61**:7–18.

McGorry PD, Goodwin RJ, Stuart GW (1988) The development, use and reliability of the Brief Psychiatric Rating Scale (Nursing Modification)—an assessment procedure for the nursing team in clinical and research settings. *Compr Psychiatry* **29**:575–587.

McGorry PD, Killackey E, Elkins K, Lambert M, Lambert T (2003) Summary Australian and New Zealand clinical guidelines for the treatment of schizophrenia. *Austral Psychiatry* **11**: 136–147.

McGorry PD, Yung AR, Phillips LJ (2001) Ethics and early intervention in psychosis: Keeping up the pace and staying in step. *Schizophr Res* **51**:17–29.

McGorry PD, Yung AR, Phillips LJ, et al (2002) Randomized controlled trial of interventions designed to reduce the risk of progression to first-episode psychosis in a clinical sample with subthreshold symptoms. *Arch Gen Psychiatry* **59**:921–928.

Miller TJ, McGlashan TH, Rosen JL, et al (2002) Prospective diagnosis of the initial prodrome for schizophrenia based on the Structured Interview for Prodromal Symptoms: Preliminary evidence of interrater and predictive validity. *Am J Psychiatry* **159**:863–865.

Miller TJ, Zipursky RB, Perkins D, et al (2003) The PRIME North America randomized double-blind clinical trial of olanzapine versus placebo in patients at risk of being prodromally symptomatic for psychosis: II Baseline characteristics of the 'prodromal' sample. *Schizophr Res;* **61**:19–30.

Miller TJ, McGlashan TH, Rosen JL, et al (in press) Prodromal assessment with the Structured Interview for Prodromal Syndromes and the Scale of Prodromal Symptoms: Predictive validity, inter-rater reliability and training to reliability. *Schizophr Bull*

Morrison AP, Bentall RP, French P, et al (2002) Randomised controlled trial of early detection and cognitive therapy for preventing transition to psychosis in high-risk individuals. Study design and interim analysis of transition rate and psychological risk factors. *Br J Psychiatry;* **43**(suppl):S78–S84.

National Early Psychosis Clinical Guidelines Working Party (2003). *Australian clinical guidelines for early psychosis.* Melbourne: University of Melbourne.

Nicholson IR, Neufeld RWJ (1992) A dynamic vulnerability perspective on stress and schizophrenia. *Am J Orthopsychiatry* **62**:117–130.

Nuechterlein KH, Dawson ME (1984) A heuristic vulnerability/stress model of schizophrenic episodes. *Schizophr Bull* **10**:300–312.

Phillips LJ, Francey SM (in press). Changing PACE: Psychological interventions in the pre-psychotic phase. In McGorry PD, Gleeson J, eds, *Psychological interventions in early psychosis: A practical treatment handbook.* Chichester, UK: Wiley.

Rogers CR, et al. (1967) *The therapeutic relationship and its impact: A study of psychotherapy with schizophrenics.* Madison: Wisconsin Press.

Sensky T, Turkington D, Kingdon D, et al (2000) A randomised controlled trial of cognitive-behavioural therapy for persistent symptoms in schizophrenia resistant to medication. *Arch Gen Psychiatry* **57**:165–172.

Wagstaff A, Perry C (2003) Clozapine: In prevention of suicide in patients with schizophrenia or schizoaffective disorder. *CNS Drugs* **17**:273–283.

Woods S, Zipursky R, Perkins D, et al (2002) Olanzapine vs. placebo for prodromal symptoms. *Acta Psychiatr Scand Suppl* **106**:43.

Woods SW, Breier A, Zipursky RB, et al (in press). Randomized trial of olanzapine vs placebo in the symptomatic acute treatment of the schizophrenic prodrome. *Biol Psychiatry*

Yung AR (2003) The schizophrenia prodrome: a high risk concept. *Schizophr Bull* **29**: 857–863.

Yung AR, McGorry PD (1996) The prodromal phase of first-episode psychosis: Past and current conceptualizations. *Schizophr Bull* **22**:353–370.

Yung AR, Phillips LJ, Yuen HP, et al (2003) Psychosis prediction: 12 month follow-up of a high risk ('prodromal') group. *Schizophr Res* **60**:21–32.

Zubin J, Spring B (1977) Vulnerability: A new view of schizophrenia. *J Abnorm Psychol* **86**:103–126.

The clinical research interface

6

The development of valid criteria for the identification of young people at heightened risk of developing a psychotic disorder has paved the way for a new era of research into the etiology of psychotic disorders, as well as the development of preventive interventions. Integration of research and clinical functions is a key element of many services but the research-clinical links are even closer in the ultra high risk (UHR) services, such as at the PACE Clinic, as this is a new type of service delivering treatment to a new patient population. There are no standardized rules or guidelines for how to manage the young people who seek help from such services. Thus, every aspect of practice within these services must be continually evaluated and modified in response to this evaluation in a constant feedback loop.

Almost all patients who attend the PACE Clinic are given the opportunity of participating in one or more of the many studies taking place within the Clinic. However, enrolling in a project is not mandatory.

When setting up a research programme involving UHR individuals, both the ethics of the research and the practicalities must be considered.

Ethics of ultra high risk (UHR) research

The following areas are relevant to UHR research, and will be discussed in turn:

- General ethical issues, pertinent to all clinical research studies involving humans.

- Issues of particular relevance to UHR research.
- Special issues unique to UHR research.

General ethical issues

Standard guidelines should always be followed when recruiting UHR individuals into research projects. These include the guiding principles of the Declaration of Helsinki: Ethical Principles for Medical Research Involving Human Subjects (first adopted by the 18th World Medical Association General Assembly, Helsinki, Finland, June 1964 with subsequent amendments—available at: http://www.wma.net/e/policy/b3.htm). Additional broad guidelines for the involvement of human participants in research are available at: http://www.nhmrc.gov.au/issues/ researchethics.htm, and http://www.nserc.ca/ programs/ethics/english/policy.htm. Pertinent considerations are outlined in Box 6.1.

Issues of particular relevance to ultra high risk (UHR) research

Recruiting minors into research

Ultra high risk (UHR) research tends to involve young people aged 14–15 years up to 25–30 years of age. Thus, a substantial number of potential research participants are aged under 18 and thus are considered to be minors under Australian law (the definition of a 'minor' may differ in other countries). Some jurisdictions will have a blanket prohibition against the inclusion of minors in research—particularly clinical trials. Others are more liberal and allow for their inclusion if a parent or guardian consents for the adolescent, usually with the adolescent providing assent. There has also been debate about adolescents' ability to consent for themselves, even in the absence of parental consent. It is argued that young people aged approximately between 14 and 18 are usually able to

Box 6.1
General ethical principles for research on humans

Informed consent
Research participants must be given sufficient information, which they clearly understand, about the research project. They must be allowed sufficient opportunity to discuss the potential involvement with those conducting the research as well as impartial independent people as considered necessary.

Separation of clinical care and research involvement
Their capacity to receive treatment should not depend on the person's decision to become involved in a research study, although their decision to be involved or not might influence the treatment they receive.

Voluntary consent
All involvement in research projects should be voluntary

Ability to withdraw consent at any time
Participants should be informed that they can withdraw their consent for participation in any research project at any time without suffering any consequences.

Confidentiality
Participants should be informed that all information they provide will be kept confidential.

understand the cost, benefits and implications of research projects and medical interventions and should be able to provide consent on their own behalf, in line with the basic ethical principle of autonomy (Beauchamp 1999). Indeed, research evidence suggests that chronological age is not the main determinant of capacity to provide informed consent (Dorn et al 1995). Another study found that 14-year-olds displayed the same level of understanding of the rationale and risk/benefit considerations of hypothetical research projects as did 21-year-olds (Weithorn 1982; Weithorn and Campbell 1982). These principles have even found their way into legal argument, with recent judgments in English courts finding that in some circumstances the consent of a parent or guardian is not essential (cited in Wing 1999). It could even be argued that it is unethical not to involve minors in research, as, under the principle of justice, they have a right to access potentially beneficial experimental treatments (Beauchamp 1999). These issues are yet to be resolved, particularly in relation to clinical trials.

Currently at the PACE Clinic, we require parental consent for minors to participate in research. We also require that the adolescent sign the consent form. Young people aged 18 years and over consent for themselves.

Informing parents of research participation

Even in the case of recruiting UHR individuals to research who are over 18 years of age, family knowledge of this involvement is always encouraged. There are many reasons for this. First, as mentioned earlier, family members are often concerned about the changes they may have noticed in the young person and want to be

involved in his or her treatment. They should be aware and informed of any research participation their family member has agreed to. Second, a family member might have questions about the research that might assist the young person in making his or her own decision about participating or not. Third, a family member might be required for aspects of the research—such as an interview about obstetric complications and early milestone development or the recruitment of siblings of UHR individuals in a magnetic resonance imaging (MRI) study. Finally, it is often useful to have a family member 'onside' to assist in encouraging the young person to keep to study protocols and so forth.

Clinical trials

Many UHR patients at the PACE Clinic, and indeed in similar UHR services around the world (see Chapter 7), receive treatment in the context of a clinical trial (McGorry et al 2003). Thus management differs from routine treatment in a purely clinical setting. Instead of a single focus on the individual patient's particular needs, clinician-researchers are concerned as well with generating reliable scientific knowledge (Carpenter et al 2003). This can lead to a potential conflict of interest for the clinician-researcher, who needs to balance these clinical and research agendas. Patients who are also research subjects may labour under what has been called the 'therapeutic misconception', that is, a belief that the research activity is meant for their direct benefit rather than to help create generalizable scientific knowledge (Wolpe et al 1999). In UHR research, the trial a patient is enrolled in often involves randomized assignment to a particular therapy, regardless of patient preferences, use of inactive placebo (considered in more detail below) and blinding of clinicians as to the exact intervention. Additionally, clinicians may be required to work within the constraints of a clinical protocol that may specify dosage levels and exclude adjunctive treatments (Carpenter et al 2003). Thus, potential subjects need to be told that there are trade-offs between a personally structured plan of care and the level of scientific rigour required in a clinical trial so they are not misled by the therapeutic misconception (Schaffner and McGorry 2001).

Use of placebo controls

Currently, there is no established treatment for either prevention of psychosis onset or for symptom management in UHR individuals. Hence, we believe it is justified to use placebo controlled designs in trials investigating treatment options. Once again, this is in line with the recommendations of the Declaration of Helsinki in which placebo controlled trials are declared ethical in the absence of existing proven therapy (http://www.wma.net/e/policy/b3.htm; Carpenter et al 2003). A clear advantage of placebo use in research trials is that a smaller sample size will probably be required to demonstrate a treatment effect than if two active medications are compared (Carpenter et al 2003; Charney et al 2002). Additionally, it must be remembered that use of placebos does not require withholding all other aspects of treatment. Psychosocial interventions, including case management, can still take place. Use of placebo can also be accompanied by a clinical plan that combines placebo with close monitoring and rapid medication intervention,

referred to as a 'clinical out' procedure, in the case of deterioration of a UHR patient. In fact, non-placebo controlled studies with a waiting list or purely monitoring arm can also present ethical challenges. Similar 'clinical outs' must be developed in these situations too, so that harm reduction can also occur in these patients.

Special issues unique to ultra high risk (UHR) research

With the rise in the pre-psychotic research, and particularly of intervention trials in this group, ethical issues associated with UHR research have attracted attention resulting in a wave of discussion and at times controversy. For example, in North America in the late 1990s complaints were made to the United States Office for Human Research Protections (OHRP) by the Citizens for Responsible Care and Research (CIRCARE) group about a randomized control trial of antipsychotic medication in a UHR group being conducted at the Yale Psychiatric Institute in the Prevention Through Risk Identification Management and Education (PRIME) Clinic (Schaffner and McGorry 2001). Amongst the group's concerns were that asymptomatic siblings of patients with schizophrenia were to be exposed to the trial and that there was no prospect of benefit to the subjects. The PRIME investigators responded to these criticisms. The first complaint is simply an error by CIRCARE. The family history ('trait') group of the PRIME Clinic is based on the same criteria developed by the PACE team, and requires not just family history in a first-degree relative, but also a significant and sustained decline in functioning.

The PRIME investigators responded to the second allegation by describing four ways in which individual subjects were likely to benefit from being involved in the trial: (1) all subjects receive monitoring of mental state; (2) all subjects receive stress management therapy; (3) those who are prescribed active medication rather than placebo are hypothesized to have a reduced risk of conversion to psychosis; and (4) those who receive active medication are likely to improve in their current symptomatology (Schaffner and McGorry 2001). These last two points have in fact been borne out by the PACE Clinic trial of antipsychotics in the UHR group (McGorry et al 2002). In this study, we found a significant reduction in rate of transition to psychosis and a decrease in symptoms and improvement in functioning for *all* patients involved (see Chapter 7 for a full description of this study). Furthermore, we believe an additional benefit to subjects is the likely rapid detection and response to psychosis in the event that a transition does occur. Hence, the duration of untreated psychosis is minimized.

There are other ethical issues particular to UHR research that must also be addressed and need to remain at the forefront of investigators' minds as further studies are developed.

Risk and prevention research

The implications of labeling a person as 'at risk' for a particular disorder have already been discussed in Chapter 4. Briefly, the issues are: stigma, changing life goals and avoiding challenges, confidentiality in relation to health insurance and employment, and the patient's potentially dysphoric reaction to such news. These issues are pertinent to UHR research as well as to clinical intervention, as reasons for research projects and subject involvement must

be explained honestly. With this in mind, the young person (and family) should be told that they are considered to have some features (either mental state changes alone, or a combination of presumed genetic risk and mental state features) that indicate an increased degree of risk of developing a psychotic disorder compared to someone from the general population. When discussing this issue, it should be emphasized that this level of risk is tempered by a number of considerations. First, the individual is symptomatic and help-seeking and has been identified as needing professional help. Second, the fact that the young person has an increased risk of psychotic disorder is coupled with the provision of a clinical service that not only provides treatment for immediate problems, but also aims to monitor the individual for signs of deterioration and intervention should a psychotic disorder become manifest. This intervention would occur without delay and hence, if psychosis does develop, the duration of untreated psychosis would be minimal. Third, general information about psychotic disorders and their treatment is also provided. Thus, the negative stereotypic image of the treatment-resistant chronic psychotic patient can be offset with more up-to-date information. This could include, for instance, information about new therapies (McGorry et al 2003), home-based treatments (Fitzgerald and Kulkarni 1998), youth-friendly services such as EPPIC (Edwards et al 2002; McGorry et al 1996) and high remission rates (Sheitman et al 1997) now known to be possible with first episode psychosis. Hence, some hope and optimism can be instilled into what may be viewed as the 'worst case scenario'—the development of frank psychosis.

Another of the difficulties in undertaking risk and preventive research is that it can never be assumed that a person declared 'at risk' will definitely develop the disorder in question (otherwise it would not be risk and prevention research, but a form of early intervention). Thus the individual receiving an intervention may not be the same individual who would develop the disorder in the absence of the intervention. Or, as Bentall and Morrison (2002) stated, 'the recipient of the benefits (the person whose illness is prevented) is not necessarily the same person as the recipient of the costs (people who may never have developed the illness but who are nonetheless exposed to the risk of side effects)' (p 352). This is true in any prevention research, not just in the present model of identifying young people at UHR of psychotic disorder. The difficulty is that we cannot distinguish between the false positives (those who were no more at risk of psychosis than someone from the general population) and the false false positives (those who would have developed a psychotic disorder had they not received some intervention) (see Chapter 3).

In the PACE Clinic we are explicit about the potential costs and benefits of research and especially intervention trials. However, the risk of a 'false positive' young person receiving treatment when they were never 'destined' to develop psychosis in the first place is offset by the clearly demonstrable benefits that UHR young people gain through treatment. All UHR patients in the PACE Clinic (false positives, false false positives and true positives), are symptomatic and help-seeking. All groups have been shown to achieve a reduction in symptomatology and improvement in functioning with intervention (McGorry et al 2002). The young people themselves generally find their treatment acceptable and helpful.

Use of antipsychotic medication in a non-psychotic group

Are antipsychotic drugs safe for those who will never really experience true psychosis? Even a little over a decade ago the response to this question would probably be 'no'. However, with the advent of safer atypical antipsychotics, with improved side-effect profiles, the cost/benefit ratio of these medications has altered (Davis et al 2003; Kapur and Remington 2001). We found a very low rate of side-effects in a UHR group treated with low dose risperidone for 6 months (McGorry et al 2002). However, longer-term side-effects of such treatment are yet to be discovered and are being investigated as part of the follow-up of this original trial cohort.

It is also unclear how long trials of treatment, both pharmacological and non-pharmacological should last. We are also unsure about the length of time UHR patients should be monitored and considered 'at risk'. This question can only be answered by further longer-term follow-up studies.

There is no question that young people who come to the attention of the PACE Clinic are experiencing substantial decreases in functioning and symptomatology (McGorry et al 2002; Yung et al 2003). Often, however, they have had difficulty obtaining support and treatment from mainstream mental health services because they do not meet criteria for a 'serious mental illness' or are not seen as 'urgent' enough (Phillips et al 1999). The development of a psychotic disorder in even 30–40% of this group of young people translates to immense personal cost and burden on the public health budget.

Reifying a new clinical entity

If UHR criteria are applied without caution then the possibility arises of over-medicalizing normal behavioural variants. This could occur, for example, if UHR criteria are applied to non-help-seeking populations, in which the base rate of psychotic disorder is very low. With any screening process, the population from which subjects are drawn is likely to affect the predictive validity of the UHR criteria. As the prevalence of a disorder decreases, so does the positive predictive value of the screening test. This is a basic epidemiological fact (Beaglehole et al 2002), the importance of which must be stressed when debating the use of the UHR criteria. Thus, if the same criteria were applied to a general population or school setting and those defined as UHR followed up for a year, the transition rate to full-blown psychosis would be a fraction of 41%. Hence, the use of these criteria should be limited to samples generated after a two or even three stage screening process. That is, the young person in question must be identified by someone in the community, or by themselves, as needing help. They must then present for help, and be identified as meeting UHR criteria. These criteria also need to be continually evaluated, and the population from which subjects are drawn taken into consideration.

Whilst working towards the development of psychosis prevention and defining an ultra high risk group, there is a risk that a new vaguely defined mental disorder, the 'at risk mental state' or 'the schizophrenic prodrome' will be created. An associated risk is that a disease model will be applied to what is essentially a heterogenous group of people with variable degrees of risk of developing psychotic symptoms of arbitrarily defined duration, frequency and intensity with variable degrees of associated disability and comorbidity. The danger is that whenever the particular UHR syndromes are seen in a young person (no matter how and where they are

noticed), well-meaning clinicians will 'diagnose' an 'at risk mental state' or 'prodrome' and start some form of treatment. This is acceptable as long as treatment is conservative. However, a problem arises when antipsychotic medication becomes the empirical first line treatment for this new 'clinical entity'. The UHR criteria should be seen as a 'work in progress' in need of continual evaluation and reflection.

Fortunately, the issues described above have not been ignored or glossed over by researchers. In fact, there is an atmosphere of openness for discussion and information sharing among researchers and a willingness to debate the issues. Discussions of the wider implications of this research are a component of regular meetings of the International Prodromal Research Network (IPRN) and other forums and have been addressed in a number of publications to date that represent all viewpoints (Bentall and Morrison, 2002; Cornblatt et al 2001; DeGrazia, 2001; Heinssen et al 2001; McGlashan, 2001; McGorry et al 2001; Schaffner and McGorry 2001; Warner, 2001; Wyatt and Henter 2001; Yung and McGorry 2003).

Practical issues in ultra high risk (UHR) research
Timing of research involvement

At the PACE Clinic, attempts are made to involve the UHR individuals in research as soon as is practicable once they are assessed and have been found to meet intake criteria. The mental state of UHR individuals often shifts rapidly and previous research has indicated that most transitions to psychosis occur within the first three months of attending the PACE Clinic (Yung et al in press). Therefore, it is essential to ensure that any baseline assessments (eg MRI scans, neuropsychological testing or niacin skin flush tests—see Chapter 7 for an explanation of these) are performed before the transition to psychosis has occurred. Recruitment to intervention studies as soon as is practicable is also desired so that potentially beneficial interventions can be commenced as soon as possible. It was earlier stated that in some cases the assessment phase can be extended to determine whether intake criteria are definitely met or not. The pressures to recruit participants to research projects should not unduly hasten the assessment phase.

Information about research studies that are underway at PACE is usually presented to the UHR individual and family members during their first or second appointment at PACE after their UHR status is confirmed. In most cases, the young people are encouraged to take some written information about research away with them to discuss with a family member or GP before the next appointment. They are then asked about their potential involvement at the next session. Such a delay between giving information and obtaining consent to participate is not always necessary depending on the size and complexity of the research project.

Introduction of research staff

It is often useful to introduce the young person and their family to all members of their treating team as well as the research staff with whom they might be in contact on a regular basis soon after their initial appointment with PACE intake staff. Introducing them to the research staff helps to put a 'human face' on research—something that might initially have frightening or worrying connotations.

Distinguishing routine clinical care from research

Of course, clinical staff are often involved in research—particularly in the case of a clinical trial. In a clinical research setting, such as the PACE Clinic, it is important that the young people taking part in research projects can differentiate between that which is routine clinical care and that which is research involvement, as well as who is involved in their treatment and who in research only. Clear explanations before gaining consent are necessary. Obviously, this is easier for some aspects of the research than others. For example, a niacin skin flush test is easily distinguished as research rather than clinical assessment. Sometimes, the distinction between research and clinical care is less obvious. For example, research staff who monitor levels of psychopathology ask many questions which overlap with clinical evaluation. It is important that UHR patients can distinguish between the two, and can be assured that information given to the researchers will not be routinely communicated to clinical staff without their consent. Thus, confidentiality is maintained. However, the young people should be warned before research interviews that under certain circumstances confidentiality cannot be guaranteed, such as when the person is suicidal or dangerous to others, in which case this information must be passed on to the treating team.

In line with the general ethical principles of research, an individual's ability to receive treatment should not be dependent on his or her decision to become involved in a research project. However, in the PACE Clinic, an individual's decision to be involved or not might influence the treatment received. For example, a young person may not wish to participate in a randomized controlled trial of low dose antipsychotic medication. At present, we do not advocate the use of antipsychotic medication in the UHR population outside of clinical trials as we believe further evaluation of its use is required. Therefore, a decision not to be involved in a trial where antipsychotic medication is an option excludes this person from this type of treatment.

Interaction between research and clinical care

Although it is important for young people taking part in research projects at PACE to be able to distinguish between research assessments and clinical care, there is also significant interaction in the Clinic between these two functions. For example, with the patient's consent, information obtained in a research interview can be shared with the treating team. This may be of great relevance for management and ensures that transition to frank psychosis, often first elicited at a research interview, is treated in a timely manner by the clinical staff. From our experience at PACE, young people rarely have a problem with information from research assessments being shared with clinicians. Indeed, they usually welcome this collaboration as it minimizes the number of times they need to tell their stories and describe their symptoms. Patients usually assent to have researchers and clinicians interview them conjointly, partly conjointly (ie with some overlap and handover of relevant information) or sequentially.

There are several other areas of potential collaboration between research and clinical functions. For example, many young people attending PACE agree to undertake neuropsychological testing as part of one of the research studies. Although the research questions that are attached to neurocognitive assessments of UHR individuals might be of primary interest to researchers, young people and their families are usually interested in the outcomes of testing and how they relate to changes they have noticed themselves, such as reduced attention, and poorer memory. Often, they request that results be forwarded to schools or other educational institutions so that teachers may best understand the difficulties they may be experiencing and how to assist with their learning. Frequently, young people are also interested in developing strategies to cope with the deficits that might be highlighted through assessment. Similarly, patients are usually interested in the results of structural brain scans. A radiologist routinely reviews these, and hence feedback can be given to the young people (usually that their brains appear normal with no overt lesions).

Issues about providing feedback to young people and their family about 'at risk' status have been discussed in an earlier chapter. Briefly, it has been the experience at PACE that this information is usually accepted well by young people and their families as long as it is provided in a constructive way that is appropriate to the level of understanding the parties have about psychosis and mental health. This includes communicating that first episode psychosis and even schizophrenia are more treatable than ever before.

Consenting procedures

International clinical guidelines for research stipulate that medical staff need to be involved in the consenting process for intervention studies/randomized controlled trials (ie MRC

Guidelines for Good Clinical Practice in Clinical Trials available at http://www.mrc.ac.uk/pdf-ctg.pdf). This also makes sense from a practical viewpoint. Young people and their families will often have questions about medication, which might be a component of a trial. Answers to such questions should come from a medical practitioner.

Consenting procedures for UHR research are linked with the information-giving process that was described in Chapter 4. The 'at risk' status should be discussed with the young people in such a manner that they understand that transition to psychosis is a possibility but not inevitable. Information about each component of a research project needs to be done explicitly. The rationale for the study, the likely benefits and potential harmful effects all need to be addressed.

Consenting to clinical trials in the UHR group is a particularly important area that has been highlighted in the literature as being associated with ethical dilemmas (Bentall and Morrison 2002). Our approach to informing potential subjects about PACE research is summarized in Box 6.2.

It has been the experience at PACE that this information is usually accepted well by young people and their families. Researchers ensure that such information is provided in a constructive way that is appropriate to the young person and the family's level of understanding about risk, psychosis and mental health.

Summary

- Young people attending the service should be given the opportunity to participate in research projects, but participation should not affect ability to access treatment.
- General and special ethical issues are involved in both providing a clinical service

Box 6.2
Content of information supplied to potential ultra high risk (UHR) research subjects

1	That it is not clear at present which form of treatment is likely to be of most benefit to them
2	That we are conducting a clinical trial to see which, if any, treatment confers most benefit to individuals who seem to be at risk of developing a psychotic disorder in the near future.
3	That the way we do this is to measure the level of people's symptoms and functioning and whether or not they develop a psychotic disorder or psychosis. Thus, we can discover which treatment or treatments confer maximum benefit.
4	In the future, such research is likely to benefit many UHR individuals who would develop a psychotic disorder in the absence of such treatment.
5	However, since the individual may or may not be truly at high risk of psychosis, the particular treatment being investigated may not have any effect on his or her chances of developing psychosis.
6	But it may be of benefit to them currently in reducing their present symptoms and improving their functioning.
7	That side-effects of trial medication may occur. These are likely to be mild and transient, and to resolve if medications are ceased.
8	That other treatment options are available, whether or not the young person consents to trial involvement, including other medications, such as antidepressants, and counselling and cognitive therapy.

to and conducting research with ultra high risk (UHR) young people.

- General principles of informed, voluntary consent, ability to withdraw consent and confidentiality apply.

- Special issues include consideration of procedures for involving minors in research, parental involvement, the cost/benefit equation in preventive research, especially taking into account the possibility of false positive status, and information giving about degree of risk.

- In practical terms, it is important to be open in consenting procedures with UHR young people and to involve their families if possible.

References

Beaglehole R, Bonita R, Kjellstrom T (2002) *Basic epidemiology*. Geneva: World Health Organization.

Beauchamp TL (1999) The philosophical basis of psychiatric ethics. In Bloch S, Chodoff P, Green SA, eds, *Psychiatric ethics* (3rd edn). Oxford University Press.

Bentall RP, Morrison AP (2002) More harm than good: The case against using antipsychotic drugs to prevent severe mental illness. *J Mental Health* 11:351–356.

Carpenter WT, Appelbaum PS, Levine RJ (2003) The declaration of Helsinki and clinical trials: A focus on placebo-controlled trials in schizophrenia. *Am J Psychiatry* 160:356–362.

Charney DS, Nemeroff CB, Lewis L, et al (2002). National depressive and manic-depressive association consensus statement on the use of placebo in clinical trials of mood disorders. *Arch Gen Psychiatry* 59:262–270.

Cornblatt BA, Lencz T, Kane JM (2001) Treatment of the schizophrenia prodrome: Is it presently ethical? *Schizophr Res* 51:31–38.

Davis JM, Chen N, Glick ID (2003) A meta-analysis of the efficacy of second-generation antipsychotics. *Arch Gen Psychiatry* 60:553–564.

DeGrazia D (2001) Ethical issues in early-intervention clinical trials involving minors at risk for schizophrenia. *Schizophr Res* 51:77–86.

Dorn LD, Susman EJ, Fletcher JC (1995) Informed consent in children and adolescents: Age, maturation and psychological state. *J Adolesc Health* 16:185–190.

Edwards J, Harris M, Herman A (2002) The Early Psychosis Prevention and Intervention Centre, Melbourne, Australia: An overview, November 2001. In Ogura C, ed, *Recent advances in early intervention and prevention in psychiatric disorders*. Tokyo: Siewa Shoten Publishers: 26–33.

Fitzgerald P, Kulkarni J (1998) Home-oriented management programme for people with early psychosis. *Br J Psychiatry;* 172(suppl):39–44.

Heinssen R, Perkins DO, Appelbaum PS, Fenton WS (2001) Informed consent in early psychosis research: National Institute of Mental Health Workshop, November 15, 2000. *Schizophr Bull* 27:571–584.

Kapur S, Remington G (2001) Atypical antipsychotics: New directions and new challenges in the treatment of schizophrenia. *Ann Rev Med* 52:503–517.

McGlashan TM (2001) Psychosis treatment prior to psychosis onset: Ethical issues. *Schizophr Res* 51:47–54.

McGorry PD, Edwards J, Mihalopolous C, et al (1996) EPPIC: An evolving system of early detection and optimal management. *Schizophr Bull* 22:305–326.

McGorry PD, Yung AR, Phillips LJ (2001). Ethics and early intervention in psychosis: Keeping up the pace and staying in step. *Schizophr Res* 51:17–29.

McGorry PD, Yung AR, Phillips LJ, et al (2002) Randomized controlled trial of interventions designed to reduce the risk of progression to first-episode psychosis in a clinical sample with subthreshold symptoms. *Arch Gen Psychiatry* 59:921–928.

McGorry P, Killackey E, Elkins K, et al (2003) Summary Australian and New Zealand clinical practice guideline for the treatment of schizophrenia (2003). *Austral Psychiatry* 11:136–147.

McGorry PD, Yung AR, Phillips LJ (2003) The 'close-in' or ultra high risk model: A safe and effective strategy for research and clinical intervention in prepsychotic mental disorder. *Schizophr Bull* 29: 771–790.

Phillips LJ, Yung AR, Hearn N, et al (1999) Preventive mental health care: Accessing the target population. *Aust NZ J Psychiatry* **33**:912–917.

Schaffner KF, McGorry PD. (2001) Preventing severe mental illnesses: New prospects and ethical challenges. *Schizophr Res* **51**:3–15.

Sheitman BB, Lee H, Strauss R, Lieberman JA (1997) The evaluation and treatment of first-episode psychosis. *Schizophr Bull* **23**:653–661.

Warner R (2001) The prevention of schizophrenia: What interventions are safe and effective? *Schizophr Bull* **27**: 551–562.

Weithorn LA (1982) Developmental factors and competence to make informed treatment decisions. *Child Youth Serv* **5**:85–100.

Weithorn LA, Campbell SB (1982) The competency of children and adolescents to make informed treatment decisions. *Child Dev* **53**:1589–1598.

Wing J (1999) Ethics and psychiatric research. In Bloch S, Chodoff P, Green SA, eds, *Psychiatric ethics* (3rd edn). Oxford University Press, 461–477.

Wolpe PR, Moreno J, Caplan AL (1999) Ethical principles and history. In Pincus HA, Lieberman JA, Feris S, eds, *Ethics in psychiatric research*. Washington DC: American Psychiatric Association, 1–21.

Wyatt RJ, Henter I (2001) Rationale for the study of early intervention. *Schizophr Res* **51**:69–76.

Yung AR, McGorry PD (2003) Keeping an open mind: Investigating options for treatment of the pre psychotic phase. *J Mental Health* **12**: 341–343.

Yung AR, Phillips LJ, Yuen HP, et al (2003) Psychosis prediction: 12 month follow-up of a high risk ('prodromal') group. *Schizophr Res* **60**:21–32.

Yung AR, Phillips LJ, Yuen HP, McGorry PD (in press). Risk factors for psychosis: Psychopathology and clinical features. *Schizophr Res*

Ultra high risk research findings

7

The last decade has seen the beginning and subsequent burgeoning of 'prodromal' or 'pre-psychotic' research in schizophrenia and related disorders. The idea was originally formulated and trialed in a population-based manner by Falloon, with a project that encouraged general practitioners in and around the English towns of Buckingham and Winslow to refer patients suspected of having a 'schizophrenic prodrome' to a mental health service for treatment. A reduction in incidence of first episode schizophrenia compared to historical figures was found and cited as possible evidence for the effectiveness of such targeted preventive intervention (Falloon et al 1990; Falloon 1992; Falloon 2000). Falloon acknowledged methodological difficulties with this approach and the fact that some people not actually at risk of schizophrenia would have been unnecessarily labelled and treated. However, this study opened the way for early intervention strategies in psychosis to consider the prodromal phase as a potential focus for treatment. The strategy has largely shifted now to the targeted approach that has been described in earlier chapters. This chapter presents some of the research to date from the PACE Clinic and other centres around the world. Broadly speaking, four areas of investigation have been conducted:

1   Validation of ultra high risk (UHR) criteria.
2   Investigations into the onset of disorder and factors that increase the likelihood of progression from 'at risk mental state' (ARMS) to psychosis.
3   Investigations into the neurobiology of psychotic disorders, especially the neurobiology of emerging psychosis.

4   The development, application and evaluation of interventions aimed at prevention, delay or amelioration of the onset of the first episode of psychosis.

These fields of research will be considered in turn.

Validation of ultra high risk (UHR) criteria

The UHR criteria and the rationale underlying their development were described in Chapter 3. The validity of these criteria has now been well supported in longitudinal studies. The first study evaluating the validity of the criteria was conducted at the PACE Clinic between 1994 and 1996. Young people meeting intake criteria were recruited and their mental state was monitored monthly over the subsequent 12 month period in order to determine the validity of the criteria for high risk of psychosis. By the end of 12 month follow-up 20 out of 49 of the subjects (41%) had developed frank psychosis and had been started on appropriate neuroleptic treatment (Yung et al 1998, 2003). This occurred despite the provision of supportive counselling, case management and antidepressant medication if required. The majority of those who developed a psychotic disorder had a DSM-IV diagnosis of schizophrenia (13 out of 20 in the psychosis group, 65%) (Yung et al 2003). The sensitivity and specificity of the criteria could not be determined as individuals who did not meet intake criteria were not followed up to determine whether they too developed psychosis.

The PACE study group was then expanded to include an additional 54 subjects, making the total sample size 104 in a subsequent publication (Yung et al in press). These 54 patients were followed up at only the 6 and 12 month time points. The transition rate in this larger sample was 27.9% (29 of 104 subjects) at 6 month follow-up and 34.6% (36 of 104) at 12 month follow-up, illustrating that the transition rate was sustained with a larger sample and with less frequent research assessments.

The at risk mental status (ARMS) concept and UHR criteria have been adopted and modified slightly by a group based at Yale University, the Prevention through Risk Identification, Management and Education (PRIME) Clinic, headed by Professor Thomas McGlashan. The PRIME group has coined the term 'Criteria of Prodromal Syndromes' (COPS) to describe their intake criteria which are based on the UHR criteria developed earlier by the PACE group. The PRIME group have also developed a semi-structured interview using the CAARMS and the Positive and Negative Symptom Scale (PANSS: Kay et al 1987) as resources, called the Structured Interview for Prodromal Syndromes (SIPS) to rate presenting symptomatology and to determine if COPS criteria are met (Miller et al 2002). Ratings are made on the Scale of Prodromal Symptoms (SOPS), also developed by the PRIME group (Miller et al in press). The PRIME investigators based their definition of the psychosis threshold on that developed at PACE, but made some changes to these criteria as well. For example, patients are considered to meet the criteria for psychosis if they have attenuated psychotic symptoms and are markedly suicidal or dangerous. The PRIME investigators followed up 14 patients who met COPS intake criteria. Using these intake and exit points, a conversion rate to psychosis of 43% (6 out of 14 subjects) at 6 months and 50% (7 of 14) at 12 month follow-up was found (Miller et al in press).

In Norway, Larsen and colleagues have used the questionnaire and criteria developed by the PRIME group to identify and follow up an ultra high risk cohort through their centre called the TOPP Clinic. Eighty-four young people have been assessed with 14 meeting COPS criteria over a two year period. Within 12 months of recruitment 6 of the 14 (43%) have developed psychosis (Larsen 2002). Similarly, the CARE programme in San Diego, USA has criteria based on those of PRIME. Latest data indicate a 16% transition rate. This relatively low rate of frank psychosis may be partly due to several patients already taking antipsychotic medication at the time of initial referral and intake into the service (Cadenhead K, email comm, September 2003).

The Early Identification and Intervention Evaluation (EDIE) trial is based in Manchester, UK. This service uses the PACE UHR intake criteria and definition of psychosis according to ratings on the PANSS (Kay et al 1987). A rate of transition to psychosis of 22% (5 of 23) over 6–12 months has been reported (Morrison et al 2002).

The Psychological Assistance Service (PAS) was established in Newcastle, Australia in 1997 and operates as a clinical service for the assessment and treatment of young people at high risk of psychosis and those experiencing a first psychotic episode. The intake criteria are based on those of PACE but also allow inclusion if a young person has a second degree relative with a history of psychotic disorder in conjunction with a significant decline in functioning (Carr et al 2000). The transition rate to psychosis, low initially, is now comparable to that of PACE, at around 50% (Schall U, pers comm 24 October 2002, Carr V, pers comm 11 August 2003).

The Portland Identification and Early Referral (PIER) service is a population-wide system of early detection that utilizes a broad ranging community education and development programme to identify individuals within the early stages of a psychotic disorder based on the COPS/UHR criteria (McFarlane et al 2002). Two definitions of conversion to psychosis are used: (1) based on the PRIME psychosis criteria; and (2) 'brief psychotic episode' defined as one day or more of frank psychotic symptoms as defined by the SIPS/SOPS (Miller et al 2002). Harm reduction intervention occurs immediately on reaching this second 'brief psychotic episode' definition of caseness, so full conversion is expected to be uncommon. The transition rates from this site compare with the experimental conditions in randomized trials in other centres using similar criteria (SIPS/SOPS). Thus, interpretation of the benefits and risks of the global intervention may be inexact, although like the Buckingham study of Falloon (Falloon 2000; Falloon et al 1990), the findings may be heuristically very useful. To date, no patients have developed a SIPS/SOPS defined psychosis, although 11 of 47 (23.4%) have developed a 'brief psychotic episode' within 12 months of follow-up. This group is now testing the psychosocial, family-based intervention system in a randomized controlled clinical trial in which medication is held constant.

At least two other centres have developed slightly different criteria to identify an 'at risk' population. The FETZ (FrühErkennungs- und Therapie Zentrum for Psychische Krisen) Centre was established in Cologne in 1997 with its own criteria for identifying the putatively prodromal population. The investigators with this Clinic are grounded in the Huberian tradition, which emphasizes the importance of 'basic symptoms' in the genesis of schizophrenia (Gross 1989; Klosterkötter 1992; Klosterkötter et al 1996) (see Chapter 3 for a detailed discussion of the basic symptoms concept). Patients attending FETZ must have experienced at least two of the following symptoms:

- Marked social withdrawal
- Marked impairment in role functioning
- Odd beliefs/magical thinking that influences behaviour and is inconsistent with cultural norms
- Ideas of reference
- Thought interference
- Pressure or perseveration of thought
- Perceptual disturbance without organic cause
- Impaired capacity to make social contact despite a desire to do so
- Increased emotional reactivity in response to everyday events.

These items are a combination of some of the DSM-III-R prodromal symptoms (American Psychiatric Association, 1987) and basic symptoms. Five of 51 individuals (9.8%) meeting these criteria developed a psychotic disorder within 15 months of follow-up (Hambrecht et al 2002).

Another different approach to identifying UHR individuals has been undertaken at the Hillside Recognition and Prevention (Hillside-RAP) programme in New York (Cornblatt et al 2002a). Investigators at this site, who bring their expertise from genetic high risk studies to the area of pre-psychotic research, have schizophrenia as their target syndrome, rather than just psychosis. Accordingly their intake and outcome criteria have been modified from the PACE and PRIME criteria. The RAP Clinic has two categories of

what are dubbed 'clinical high risk ' (CHR) patients. This terminology is used to contrast these putatively prodromal individuals from subjects recruited through the traditional high risk projects which use family history as the sole intake criterion [ie New York High Risk Project: (Erlenmeyer-Kimling et al 1995), the Copenhagen High Risk Project (Cannon and Mednick 1993) and the Israeli High Risk Study (Ingraham et al 1995)]. The two intake groups in the RAP Clinic are: (1) the clinical high risk (CHR$^+$) (positive) group, which consists of adolescents with attenuated positive psychotic symptoms (according to SIPS scores); and (2) the CHR$^-$ (negative) group, which includes young people displaying specific combinations of Cognitive, Academic and Social Impairments and Disorganization/odd behaviour (CASID features: Cornblatt et al 2002a). The CHR$^-$ group are thought to be at heightened risk of developing schizophrenia because of cognitive impairments, which are thought to precede the onset of schizophrenia. Specific operationalized criteria for identifying the CHR$^-$ group have not yet been published. The RAP investigators hypothesize that the developmental course of schizophrenia follows a progression from CHR$^-$ to CHR$^+$ to 'schizophrenia-like psychosis' (SLP: essentially schizophreniform/brief psychotic disorder) to schizophrenia. The transition rate from CHR$^+$ status to psychotic disorder, using both the PACE and PRIME Clinics' definitions of psychosis, was 26.5% (9 of 34 patients) within 6 months (Lencz et al in press), a rate similar to the 6 month transition rate in the PACE Clinic (Yung et al 2003). The transition rate to schizophrenia in the SLP's group was 33% (Cornblatt et al 2002b).

Table 7.1 summarizes the rates of transition to frank psychosis from the various UHR clinics around the world.

Table 7.1
Comparison of different rates of transition to psychosis in different ultra high risk (UHR) centres

UHR centre	Intake criteria	Psychosis criteria	No. in sample	No. and (%) psychotic within 12 months
PACE	PACE UHR criteria	PACE psychosis criteria	104	36 (34.6)
PRIME	PRIME COPS criteria	PRIME psychosis criteria	14	7 (50)
TOPP	Based on PRIME COPS criteria	Based on PRIME psychosis criteria	14	6 (43)
CARE	Based on PRIME COPS criteria	Based on PRIME psychosis criteria	25	4 (16)
EDIE	Based on PACE UHR criteria	Based on PACE psychosis criteria	23	5 (22)
PAS	Based on PACE UHR criteria, but with addition of family history of psychotic disorder in second degree relatives	Based on PACE psychosis criteria	74	37 (50)[1]
PIER	Based on PRIME COPS criteria	1. PRIME psychosis criteria 2. One day or more of frank psychotic sys	47	11 (23.4)
FETZ	FETZ criteria	Acute psychosis	51	5 (9.8) over 15 months
RAP	RAP CHR⁺ criteria	PACE and PRIME psychosis criteria	34	9 (26.5)

[1]PAS follow-up period is for longer than 12 months, and can vary between subjects.

It must be remembered when evaluating the rates of transition to psychosis in each of these centres, that the population from which subjects are drawn is likely to affect the predictive validity of the intake (UHR) criteria. As the prevalence of a disorder decreases, the positive predictive value decreases also (Mojabai et al in press). Thus, if the same UHR criteria were applied to a general population or school setting and those defined as UHR followed up for a year, the transition rate to full-blown psychosis would be much less than 41%, depending on the base rate of psychotic disorder in the population. Thus, the criteria need to be continually evaluated, and the population from which subjects are drawn taken into consideration.

Additionally, the UHR criterion of *help-seeking* must be highlighted. The UHR criteria in the original PACE study, and all subsequent studies in the PACE Clinic, were applied to a help-seeking population. That is, the young people, or others close to them, recognized that they were having problems and referred them to a service for care. They were sufficiently disturbed or distressed to warrant some kind of clinical attention, for example from a general practitioner or family doctor, a counselling service, or even a mental health service, from whence they were referred to the PACE Clinic. The UHR criteria have not been evaluated in a non-help-seeking population. We do not know what the transition rate to psychosis would be in non-help seekers who otherwise meet the criteria. This is particularly pertinent in the light of several population studies that have reported large numbers of people with attenuated psychotic symptoms and 'psychotic-like experiences' who were not distressed by their experiences and did not seek help (Eaton et al 1991; Peters et al 1999a,b; Tien 1991; van Os et al 2000, 2001).

Identification of factors associated with psychosis onset in the ultra high risk (UHR) group

In addition to establishing the validity of the UHR criteria, efforts have been made to identify features that differentiate between UHR patients who develop a psychotic episode and those who do not.

Psychopathology

One major area of research at the PACE Clinic has been the investigation of the predictive power for psychosis onset of certain mental state and illness variables. A transition rate to psychosis of 41% was found in a cohort of 49 UHR young people recruited to PACE between 1994 and 1996 (Yung et al 1998, 2003). The predictive validity of a range of mental state features at intake to the study was assessed and some highly significant predictors of psychosis were found over and above ARMS criteria. This study was recently extended with a larger cohort of 104 UHR young people (Yung et al in press). Again, some highly significant predictors of psychosis were found, which are shown in Box 7.1.

In this sample of 104 UHR young people, we examined dichotomized versions of those variables that were highly predictive of psychosis. These were: belonging to both the Trait and Attenuated Groups, duration of symptoms greater than 1825 days (5 years), GAF score less than 40 and SANS attention score greater than 2. We then examined the predictive power of

Box 7.1
Mental state features at intake predicting onset of psychosis in the ultra high risk (UHR) cohort

- Long duration of psychiatric symptoms prior to attending PACE
- Poor functioning at intake (assessed using the Global Assessment of Functioning: American Psychiatric Association 1994)
- Being a member of both the Family history (Trait) and Attenuated Symptom groups
- Depression (according to the Hamilton Rating Scale for Depression (Hamilton 1960))
- Disorganization (according to the score on the Attention subscale of the Scale for the Assessment of Negative Symptoms (Andreasen 1982)).

having one or more of these 4 'predictive factors'. Table 7.2 shows the data associated with this model for development of psychosis within 12 months.

The specificity, positive predictive value and negative predictive value of this model were all high (92.6%, 80.8%, 81.8%, respectively) and the sensitivity moderate (58.3%). The positive predictive value (PPV) is possibly the most useful of these parameters from a clinical perspective as it indicates the proportion of people with a positive test result (in this case having one or more of the predictive factors) who actually develop the disorder (in this case psychosis). The PPV of this model suggests that if a young person who attends PACE and meets the UHR criteria has any one (or more) of the predictive factors at the time of beginning intake to the clinic, then he or she has over 80% risk of developing psychosis within one year. This is an important finding that needs to be replicated. In particular, this model needs to be applied to other samples of UHR patients distinct from the sample which generated the model in order to truly test its predictive power. If this finding can

be repeated then there are clinical ramifications. Should the person be told about this degree of risk? Does this justify use of antipsychotic medication? These are ongoing questions that need further thought and investigation.

Substance use

Whilst the young people attending the PACE Clinic are advised not to use drugs and counselling strategies such as motivational interviewing (Miller and Rollnick 1991) are employed to encourage a review of drug use, the use of illicit substances, such as cannabis, LSD, Ecstasy and volatile substances, is closely monitored in young people attending the PACE Clinic. This enables the role these substances play in the onset of disorder to be assessed. Psychotic symptoms are known to occur in many individuals after using cannabis (Tart 1970; Thomas 1993; Tien and Anthony 1990), LSD and other hallucinogens (Strassman 1984) and other illicit substances, such as Ecstasy (3,4-methylenedioxymetamphetamine or MDMA: Steele et al 1994), other

Table 7.2
Psychosis status at 12 month follow-up compared to presence or absence of at least one 'predictive factor'[1] at baseline

	Psychosis within 12 months	No psychosis within 12 months	Total
One or more 'predictive factor' present	21	5	26
No 'predictive factor' present	14	63	77
Total	36	68	103[2]

[1]'Predictive factors' are: belonging to both the Trait and Attenuated Groups, duration of symptoms >1825 days (5 years), GAF score <40 and SANS attention score >2.
[2]A GAF score was missing for one subject, hence calculations are based on a sample of 103.

amphetamines: (Hall and Hando 1994) and cocaine (Satel et al 1991), but their exact role in the onset of *disorder* is less clear. Interestingly, drug use in UHR individuals attending PACE, is relatively low compared to early psychosis cohorts reported elsewhere (King et al 1994; Kovasznay et al 1997; Linszen et al 1994; Rabinowitz et al 1998).

The role of cannabis in the onset of psychosis was assessed in the PACE Clinic. Contrary to expectations, neither cannabis use nor dependence in the year prior to contact with the PACE Clinic was associated with a higher risk of developing psychosis over the following year (Phillips et al 2002a). This was surprising, given the association between cannabis use and increased likelihood of psychotic relapse described in the literature (Cuffel and Chase 1994; Linszen et al 1994). Firm conclusions about the role of cannabis in psychosis onset cannot be drawn from our data, however, because of the relatively low use of substances, including cannabis, when compared to the general population (Phillips et al 2002a). This may be due to the PACE sample including mainly help-seeking individuals, who may not be typical of the whole population of people at risk of psychosis. Individuals with high levels of cannabis use may well be less highly motivated to seek treatment than our subjects. Hence, our research is biased against finding cannabis as a risk factor for psychosis. Additionally, we were able to report analysis of cannabis use at intake only. Changes in cannabis use over the study period were therefore not picked up, and these may have been important in influencing psychosis onset (Yung et al in press). While this study did not support a role for cannabis in the development of first episode psychosis, it is too early to rule it out completely as a candidate risk factor. So far, no other studies

have produced results of investigations of the role of cannabis in the development of acute psychosis from an ARMS.

The role of other substances in the development of acute psychosis among PACE UHR individuals has not yet been investigated, as their levels of use are too low.

Stress

The ability to identify individuals at high risk of developing a psychotic disorder and the capacity to follow them through time also allows the potential role of stress in the onset of disorder to be assessed. Both physiological and psychological aspects of stress can be analysed.

The hypothalamic-pituitary-adrenal (HPA) axis is one of the primary systems moderating the physiological response to stressors—both psychological and physical (O'Brien 1997; Sapolsky et al 2000). Cortisol is one of the hormones that is involved in this process. It has been suggested that impaired HPA axis functioning might mediate between stress and the onset and course of psychotic disorders. This hypothesis is supported by reports of higher cortisol levels (plasma, salivary or urinary) and abnormal circadian cortisol levels in individuals with schizophrenia compared to healthy control subjects (eg Altamura et al 1989; Kaneko et al 1992; Lammers et al 1995; Meltzer et al 2001; Mück-Seler et al 1999). Additionally, individuals with schizophrenia have been reported to have lower urinary cortisol levels than patients with bipolar disorder (manic phase) and major depressive disorder (Yehuda et al 1990) and significantly lower numbers of glucocorticoid receptors (GR) than patients with post-traumatic stress disorder (PTSD) and bipolar (mania) (Yehuda et al

1993). Patients with schizophrenia have also been found to have higher levels of dexamethasone suppression test (DST) non-suppression than healthy controls and lower levels than depressed patients (Yeragani 1990). It is hypothesized that abnormal HPA axis responses to stress might result in hippocampal damage as this brain region is one area of the brain intimately involved in the stress response. This might then compromise attention, memory and other cognitive skills and ultimately influence the development of psychotic symptoms such as delusional thoughts, hallucinations and thought disorder (Figure 7.1). This model draws together many of the putative vulnerability markers that are described above and stress/distress.

Monitoring cortisol levels can assess HPA axis functioning. In the PACE cohort this is done by obtaining salivary and plasma cortisol levels at

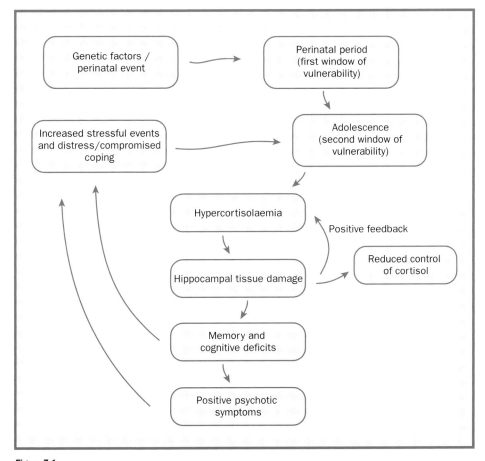

Figure 7.1
Stress and psychosis model.

baseline and monthly salivary samples for 12 months or until acute psychosis develops. Samples are all obtained at 8 am. Any rises in cortisol level over time that might be associated with increased level of distress or anxiety preceding the acute onset can then be assessed.

A pilot project has been conducted at PACE to assess this hypothesis. The results of this study did not demonstrate a relationship between cortisol levels at baseline and later development of psychosis in a UHR cohort. The number of participants in this study was very small, however (*n* = 27), with only 11% developing psychosis within 12 months. A larger study is currently underway at the PACE Clinic.

Studies of the relationship between the experience of stress from a psychological perspective and the onset and course of psychotic disorders, particularly schizophrenia, have been ongoing for many years. Evidence in support of this proposed association is far from compelling. Many studies, including the seminal study by Brown and Birley (1968) have indicated that the level of stress increases prior to the onset of a psychotic episode or a relapse (Canton and Fraccon, 1985; Mazure et al 1997; Schwartz and Myers 1977). Other studies have failed to show such a relationship (Chung et al 1986; Clancy et al 1973; Gruen and Baron 1984; Jacobs and Myers, 1976; Malzacher et al 1981). There is much stronger evidence to suggest that individuals with psychotic disorders have compromised coping skills compared to healthy individuals. (van den Bosch et al 1992; Jansen et al 1999). A study is currently taking place at PACE to assess whether UHR individuals who develop frank psychosis experience heightened levels of stressors and cope with stress differently compared to UHR individuals who do not develop psychosis and healthy controls.

The neurobiology of psychosis onset

Brain imaging

The most commonly accepted etiopathological model of schizophrenia is the neurodevelopmental theory (Murray and Lewis 1987; Weinberger 1987). This model proposes that abnormalities in fetal brain development underlie the pathogenesis of schizophrenia. This theory seems to have arisen as a response to the fact that almost no neuropathological evidence for necrotic neurodegeneration in schizophrenia could be found in post-mortem studies of the brains of people with schizophrenia (Harrison and Roberts 2000), with the absence of gliosis being thought of as evidence for the timing of the pathological process in the early stage of brain development when no inflammatory reactions can take place. In fact, the lack of gliosis only demonstrates that *necrotic* cell death (as opposed to apoptosis) is not substantially involved in the pathogenesis of onset and course of schizophrenia.

The neurodevelopmental model gained some currency when several studies found neuroimaging anomalies in first episode samples (see reviews by Pantelis et al 2003a; Velakoulis et al 1999). Because the first episode patients were considered to be in the phase close to the 'onset' of the disorder, these brain abnormalities were said to have been present prior to disorder onset. Thus these studies were interpreted as supportive of a static structural abnormality associated with schizophrenia, which had originated early in neurodevelopment (Shenton et al 2001). The problem with this reasoning is that the first episode of psychosis may not reflect onset of schizophrenia at all, but may in fact be a late manifestation of some underlying brain pathology. It may be that onset of the prodrome, or some other point lying between the beginning of the prodrome (a very ill-defined point, as discussed in Chapter 3) and the onset of frank psychosis (another ill-defined point) may be a more accurate indicator of the onset of illness and neurological malfunction.

Challenging the neurodevelopmental model of schizophrenia are post-mortem studies which demonstrate anomalies of cortical lamination, and neuronal positioning that could be explained in the context of a potentially biologically active process that might be relevant during adolescence and early adulthood (Harrison and Roberts 2000). In addition, more recent post-mortem evidence suggests a reduction in number of glial cells in the brains of patients with schizophrenia (Cotter et al 2001; Coyle and Schwarcz 2000), the timing of which is unclear.

The alternative to the neurodevelopmental theory, the neurodegenerative hypothesis, postulates that neurological abnormalities emerge later, around the time of the first clinical manifestations of the illness, which, as noted above, could be conceptualized as either around the time of the onset of the prodrome or around the time of onset of frank positive psychotic symptoms, or some point between the two. It may be that in at least some patients neurological abnormalities are present pre- or perinatally, and then further brain changes occur later in the course of illness. We could speculate, for example, that the loss of glial cells may occur around the time of the first clinical manifestations of schizophrenia and may play a part in the triggering of onset.

Investigations of UHR individuals provide the opportunity to investigate whether or not brain abnormalities are present prior to the onset of frank psychosis. The UHR methodology

cannot, however, shed light on whether changes occur around the time of prodrome onset, as patients are already symptomatic and putatively prodromal at the time of entry to the Clinic. The target brain areas to study are the hippocampus and other temporal lobe structures (Pantelis et al 2003a; Velakoulis et al 1999), regions that have been found to be the location of many brain abnormalities in schizophrenia.

Consistent with the neurodevelopmental hypothesis, hippocampal volumes of PACE UHR patients at intake lie midway between those of normal controls and patients with chronic schizophrenia or first episode psychosis (Phillips et al 2002b). Also compared with healthy controls, male UHR subjects are less likely to have a well-developed left para-cingulate gyrus and more likely to have interruptions in the course of the left cingulate septum (Yücel et al 2003). These latter findings mirror results of similar studies in patients with established psychotic disorders (Yücel et al 2003).

When the UHR cohort is divided into those who became psychotic within 12 months and those who did not, cross-sectional comparisons show that the UHR individuals who subsequently developed psychosis had significantly smaller grey matter volumes in the right medial temporal region, including the hippocampus and para-hippocampal cortex (Pantelis et al 2003b). Other brain regions that differed in volume between UHR individuals who later developed psychosis and those who did not included a right lateral temporal region (including superior temporal gyrus and temporal region), a right inferior frontal region (including orbital portion of inferior frontal gyrus and adjacent parts of the insula and basal ganglia) and a cingulate region (incorporating the anterior and posterior cingulate gyrus bilaterally)

(Pantelis et al 2003b). Morphology of the paracingulate gyrus and cingulate sulcus did not differentiate between those UHR individuals who later developed psychosis and those who did not (Yücel et al 2003).

However, against the neurodevelopmental model, reduced hippocampal volumes in the UHR cohort at baseline have not been shown to be associated with a heightened risk of later developing acute psychosis. In fact, those UHR patients with larger (although in the normal range) left hippocampal volumes at intake were more likely to develop a psychotic episode in the subsequent 12 month period (Phillips et al 2002b). This was due to the UHR subjects who did not develop psychosis (the false positives) in fact having smaller than average hippocampal volumes. It must be remembered that these false positives are not normal healthy controls. They are help-seeking and symptomatic with a range of symptoms and psychiatric syndromes (see Chapter 5 for more detail). The reduced hippocampal volume in this subsample of patients may reflect this non-psychotic psychopathology.

In a subsample of UHR patients who developed psychosis, we obtained magnetic resonance imaging (MRI) brain scans at baseline (ie prior to onset of frank psychosis) and one year later (post psychosis). Scans showed a significant bilateral reduction in grey matter volume in the cingulate region as well as in the left para-hippocampal gyrus, left fusiform gyrus, left orbitofrontal cortex and one region of the left cerebellar cortex (Pantelis et al 2003b). These findings were not present in a group of UHR patients scanned at baseline and one year later but who did not develop psychosis. This exciting finding suggests that brain changes can occur during the process of transition to psychosis,

and, while the basis of this remains uncertain, opens up the possibility that with sufficiently early treatment such changes could be minimized or aborted.

In addition to obtaining MRI brain scans of the PACE UHR young people, proton magnetic resonance imaging (^{1}H MRS) of the left medial temporal and left dorsolateral prefrontal regions has also been obtained on 30 UHR clients and results compared with MRS of 56 first episode psychosis patients and 21 healthy controls. Twenty per cent of this UHR cohort developed psychosis within 12 months of the scan. No differences were identified between the first episode and control groups for any metabolite ratio in either region-of-interest, possibly indicating intact neuronal circuitry in the early phase of psychotic disorders. Similarly, there were no differences between the UHR and control groups for the medial temporal region. A significant elevation of the *N*-acetyl-aspartate (NAA)/creatine and the choline/creatine ratios in the dorsolateral prefrontal region of the UHR group was found compared to the healthy comparison group. This finding did not differentiate between those UHR individuals who later became psychotic and those who did not. This could be interpreted as a decline in creatine, indicative of hypometabolism, and provides a possible explanation for the poorer working memory of UHR patients (Wood et al, in press).

To date, there have been no other reports of studies using brain imaging in other UHR cohorts.

Olfactory identification

Assessments of olfactory (smell) identification ability provide an indication of circuitry involving the orbitofrontal cortex. Deficits in olfactory identification are consistently found in patients with chronic schizophrenia (Brewer et al 1996) and first episode psychosis (Brewer et al 2001; Moberg et al 1997; Seidman et al 1997). We examined the olfactory identification ability in the UHR group in order to discover whether these impairments were present before psychosis onset and whether they had any predictive power in relation to psychosis onset. The olfactory identification ability of 81 PACE UHR individuals was compared to 31 healthy comparison subjects. Twenty-two of the UHR patients (27.2%) later became psychotic. Those UHR individuals who later developed a schizophrenia spectrum disorder (12 members of the cohort) displayed a significant impairment in olfactory identification ability compared to the UHR individuals who did not develop psychosis, the UHR individuals who developed a non-schizophrenia spectrum disorder and the healthy comparison group. These findings could suggest that the incipient onset of schizophrenia compromises normal frontal lobe development and therefore interferes with the development of neuropsychological functions mediated by these regions. Thus olfactory identification impairment might be a premorbid marker of transition to schizophrenia, but may not be predictive of psychotic illness more generally (Brewer et al 2003). However, this is speculative and thus far based on research in a small sample. Replication in a larger study group is needed.

Neurocognitive assessments

Although not central to the diagnosis, cognitive impairment is common in schizophrenia. Specifically, individuals with schizophrenia have been found to have poorer memory, executive functioning skills (planning, cognitive flexibility, abstract thinking and information processing) and attention skills than non-affected individuals (Heinrichs and Zakzanis 1998). Certain neurocognitive deficits, such as attention, have been proposed as vulnerability markers for schizophrenia although most have not yet been adequately validated (Kremen et al 1994; Wolf and Cornblatt 1996). Longitudinal assessment of cognitive functions in UHR individuals provides an opportunity to assess whether these deficits predate the onset of psychosis (vulnerability marker) or whether they come 'online' once acute psychosis has developed (Cadenhead, 2002).

Particular interest has been paid to the Continuous Performance Task (CPT), an assessment of attention (Cornblatt et al 1988). As indicated above, attention has been highlighted as impaired in individuals with schizophrenia (Heinrichs and Zakzanis 1998). It has also been suggested that impaired attention might be a vulnerability marker for later development of schizophrenia (Michie et al 2000; Nuechterlein and Dawson 1984). Results to date at PACE have indicated that the performance of PACE UHR individuals on the CPT indicating attentional capacity lay between healthy control subjects and first episode psychosis patients but was closer to the performance of the first episode group (Francey 2002). No differences were found on performance on the CPT at baseline between UHR individuals who later developed psychosis and those who did not (Francey 2002).

The performance of UHR individuals attending the PACE Clinic on a range of other neurocognitive tests has been compared with individuals with established or first episode psychosis as well as healthy age-matched controls. UHR individuals showed marked impairments in performance on tests of spatial working memory and delayed matching to sample than a healthy comparison group. The UHR individuals who later developed psychosis generally performed more poorly than those who did not on these tasks, although this did not reach significance for any measure. Further investigation is required to assess the validity of working memory as a predictive tool for psychosis (Wood et al 2003).

PACE UHR subjects have also been found to show significantly worse performance on the Performance and Full (short-form) IQ scales of the WAIS-R (Ward 1990; Wechsler, 1981) compared to controls. In addition, impairment has also been found in measures of visual recall, and the Verbal Memory Index of the Weschler Memory Scale – Revised (WMS-R) although these differences were not significant (Brewer et al, in prep). More interesting is the finding that there are some differences at baseline between those UHR young people who eventually develop psychosis compared to those who do not. The group that made the transition to psychosis performed significantly more poorly than the group that did not on tests of logical memory and the Visual Reproduction test. Both these tests essentially require the rapid processing of incoming information and efficiently organizing it for accurate recall. In addition, both are unstructured in the manner in which recall is initiated. This suggests that the application of efficient organizational strategies is compromised at baseline in the UHR group which develop psychosis later (Brewer et al in prep). This finding is suggestive of prefrontal impairments. This is in accordance with our findings of impaired spatial working memory

(Wood et al 2003), poorer olfactory identification (Brewer et al 2003) and lower frontal grey matter volumes (Pantelis et al 2003b) in this population.

The only other centres that have investigated neurocognitive functioning of UHR individuals are the PRIME Clinic and FETZ. The performance of young people attending the PRIME Clinic and meeting COPS criteria on a range of neurocognitive tests assessing intellectual functioning, memory, executive functioning and attention was intermediate to normal controls and schizophrenia samples (Hawkins et al 2003). The UHR group seen at FETZ who met their unique intake criteria performed worse than healthy controls on tests of verbal fluency, attention and memory function (Hambrecht et al 2002).

Obstetric complications

In line with the neurodevelopmental model of psychotic disorders, it is thought that early life trauma, such as obstetric complications, might impact on brain development resulting in a vulnerability to later psychotic illness (Geddes and Lawrie 1995a,b; McNeil and Cantor-Graae 2000). At PACE, an interview is conducted with the parents of the UHR young people to assess the occurrence of obstetric complications and the achievement of childhood milestones. A semi-structured interview called the Childhood Developmental Risk Factor Index, which combines items from the Lewis-Murray obstetric complications scale (Lewis and Murray 1987), and the Premorbid Adjustment Scale (Cannon-Spoor et al 1982), is used to assess these factors. To date, although UHR individuals experienced more childhood traumatic events than healthy control subjects and had a higher level of schizotypal and schizoid traits, these factors were not associated with a higher risk of developing frank psychosis. In fact, the UHR group achieved childhood milestones earlier on average than a control group, but this also was not associated with a higher chance of becoming psychotic. No differences were found between the groups in the frequency of a range of obstetric complications. Once again, limitations with this study, including small sample size, suggest that it is too early to completely dismiss obstetric complications as playing a role in the vulnerability towards later psychotic disorder. Results from other centres that have investigated this putative risk factor are keenly awaited.

Altered membrane lipid chemistry

There is some support for the theory that membrane lipid chemistry is altered in some patients with schizophrenia (Berger et al 2002). Some evidence for this comes from a test that examines skin sensitivity to niacin. The normal response to topical application of niacin is flushing of the skin, a reaction which is mediated by prostaglandins which themselves derive from arachidonic acid (AA), one of the main bioactive lipids of the brain and precursor of many second messengers. It has been hypothesized that the AA-prostaglandin second messenger pathway might be altered in patients with schizophrenia. In support of this theory is the finding that the skin flush reaction to niacin is markedly reduced or absent in patients with schizophrenia compared to healthy controls (Hudson et al 1997; Shah et al 2000; Ward et al 1998). In addition, reduced AA levels have been found in the cell membranes of some individuals with schizophrenia (Horrobin et al 1991; Yao et al 2000).

Our group has developed a new semi-quantitative, descriptive assessment scale for the niacin skin flush test, which provides a valid and reliable measure to assess niacin sensitivity. Using this methodology, we found that about 40–50% of first episode psychosis patients have impaired niacin skin reaction compared to normal controls. Further, it is hypothesized that the insensitivity to topical niacin might be a biological marker for future development of psychosis, in at least a subgroup of patients. We are currently investigating this possibility by performing the niacin skin flush test on UHR individuals at 3 monthly intervals at the PACE Clinic. Results are pending.

Viruses

It has been proposed that psychosis in at least some cases might be the result of viral central nervous system (CNS) infections (Torrey 1988; Yolken and Torrey 1995). This hypothesis is based on the association of psychotic symptoms with some viral encephalitides, and epidemiological studies of the prevalence of maternal infections during pregnancy in schizophrenia (Brown et al 2000). CNS infection could either be due to primary infection or to the reactivation of organisms that were originally acquired earlier in life. Several lines of evidence suggest that inflammatory and/or immunological mechanisms are involved in the etiology of schizophrenia and other psychoses. First, the non-specific immune system shows signs of an overactivation in unmedicated schizophrenic patients, indicated by increased counts of monocytes and gamma delta-cells. Second, increased levels of interleukin-6 (IL-6) and the activation of the IL-6 system in schizophrenia might also be the result of the activation of monocytes/macrophages. Finally, impairment of the blood-cerebrospinal fluid barrier which has been observed in patients with schizophrenia has been linked to vascular leakage due to an inflammatory process (Hart et al 1999; Lin et al 1988; Müller et al 1999; Nikkila et al 1999; Rapaport and Lohr 1994; Schwarz et al 1998). However, the research investigating a possible role of infectious agents in schizophrenia and other neuropsychiatric disorders is controversial.

Many studies have been published investigating the role of herpes viruses (herpes simplex virus type 1, cytomegalovirus, Epstein-Barr virus, varicella-zoster virus and herpes virus type 6), Borna disease virus and other viruses, such as measles, rubella, mumps, influenza A and B, and retroviruses in schizophrenia (eg Alexander et al 1992; Carter et al 1987; Conejero-Goldberg et al 2003; de Lisi et al 1986; Hart et al 1999; Karlsson et al 2001; Srikanth et al 1994). Most studies have applied serum antibodies against infectious agents as a method to detect CNS infection. Others have investigated cerebral spinal fluid, brain tissue, or both. Altogether, results are inconsistent, with about half of the studies failing to find positive associations, according to a review by O'Reilly (1994). Additionally, these studies have methodological limitations. The UHR patient group provides an ideal population within which to further assess this possible causal relationship. At the PACE Clinic we are investigating the role of viruses in the onset of psychotic disorders by analysing blood samples of UHR young people at initial contact with the Clinic for a range of viral antibodies.

Treatment studies

Intervention studies in ultra high risk (UHR) cohorts with a view to developing preventive interventions are in their infancy. Validation of the criteria for identifying individuals at ultra high risk of psychosis has been viewed as an important first step to ensure that treatment is provided to appropriate individuals whilst minimizing those who receive treatment unnecessarily. Thus, appropriately, intervention studies have lagged behind the validation studies.

Antipsychotic medication

The first randomized controlled trial specifically developed around the needs of the UHR population with the aim of preventing, delaying or ameliorating the onset of psychosis, was conducted at the PACE Clinic from 1996 to 1999 (McGorry et al 2002). This was described in detail in Chapter 5. Essentially, the impact of intensive cognitive-behaviour oriented psychotherapy plus low dose neuroleptic (risperidone) was compared with the effect of supportive therapy alone on the development of illness in the UHR group. There was a significantly higher rate of transition to psychosis in the control (supportive therapy) group ($n = 28$) compared to the intervention group ($n = 31$) at the end of the 6 month treatment phase ($p = .026$). This difference was no longer significant at the 12 month follow-up point. This result is thought to indicate a delay in the onset of psychosis in the intervention group. Both groups experienced a reduction in global psychopathology and functioning over the treatment phase (McGorry et al 2002). Longer-term follow-up of the participants in this study is now taking place. A second randomized trial is also currently underway at PACE. In this second study, the treatment phase has been extended to 12 months, the psychological treatment component has been modified and strengthened, and a three cell design is employed: low dose antipsychotic medication plus cognitive therapy, placebo plus cognitive therapy, and placebo alone. Additionally, the research team and participants are blind to group membership.

Preliminary results of the first randomized controlled trial (RCT) at the PRIME Clinic also indicate that UHR patients benefit from the provision of specific antipsychotic treatment, in this case olanzapine (McGlashan et al 2003; Miller et al 2003; Woods et al in press). Thirty UHR patients who received olanzapine reported lower levels of 'prodromal' symptomatology, according to the SIPS (Miller et al 2002), after 8 weeks of treatment compared to 29 UHR patients who received placebo medication. After 12 months of treatment, the group that received olanzapine had a significant reduction in psychotic ('prodromal') symptomatology whereas the placebo group did not. There was also a lower transition rate to psychosis in the olanzapine group than the placebo group after 12 months of treatment (McGlashan et al 2002).

Antidepressants

Cornblatt and colleagues (2002a) argued that antidepressant medication should be considered as a possible preventive intervention. This suggestion is based on results of a 'naturalistic' treatment study in New York, which surveyed the type of treatment offered to young people meeting intake criteria for the RAP Clinic. No direction was given to medical practitioners regarding the treatment they should provide for UHR individuals. The researchers were interested in what line of treatments were commonly offered to assist the young people with the range of difficulties and symptoms they presented with. Over 80% of patients received a

pharmacological treatment with the remainder receiving psychotherapy. The latter was restricted to the CHR⁻ (clinical high risk negative) group whereas all of those in the SLP group received an antipsychotic medication. Members of the CHR⁺ and CHR⁻ groups who were treated with medication received either antipsychotic medication or an antidepressant with both demonstrating clinical improvements (Cornblatt et al 2002a). It is noted that 41.9% of the intervention group and 60.7% of the control group in the first RCT at the PACE Clinic were prescribed an antidepressant medication (McGorry et al 2002).

Lithium

Recent research has suggested that lithium at low doses has a neurotrophic or neuroprotective effect that is mediated through the increased production of the enzyme bcl-2 in response to lithium in rat (Manji et al 2000a) and human brains (Manji et al 1999). Bcl-2 is widely regarded as a major neuroprotective protein and increased bcl-2 levels have demonstrated not only robust protection of neurons against diverse insults but have also demonstrated an increase in regeneration of mammalian CNS axons. Post-mortem temporal cortex of schizophrenic, bipolar, and depressed subjects showed a 25% reduction of bcl-2 protein compared to normal controls (Jarskog et al 2000). A secondary analysis of schizophrenic and bipolar subjects revealed twofold higher mean bcl-2 concentrations in antipsychotic-treated versus neuroleptic-naive subjects. Less bcl-2 protein in the untreated patients may signal neuronal vulnerability to both pro-apoptotic stimuli and neuronal atrophy. The association between neuroleptic exposure and higher bcl-2 levels could underlie the favourable long-term outcomes of patients who receive maintenance antipsychotic treatment.

Lithium also has been shown to be associated with a range of other effects that impact on the process of apoptosis (neuronal cell death) and its suppressive effects on mRNA expression and protein transcription of pro-apoptotic p53 (Manji et al 2000b).

Neuropathological and neuroimaging studies suggest neuronal dysfunction in schizophrenia. To date, the most consistently replicated spectroscopic finding in schizophrenia is reduced *N*-acetyl-aspartate (NAA) levels in the hippocampal and prefrontal regions, obtained through [1]H-magnetic resonance spectroscopy (^{1}H-MRS) (Block et al 2000; Vance et al 1999; Weinberger 1999). Since NAA is thought to be a marker for neuronal/axonal integrity, NAA reductions have been interpreted as strong evidence for neuronal/axonal loss or dysfunction in these brain regions.

After 4 weeks of lithium treatment at therapeutic levels an increase in total brain NAA concentration ($p < .0217$) (Moore et al 2000) could be demonstrated using ^{1}H-MRS in medication-free bipolar patients and healthy volunteers in frontal, temporal, parietal, and occipital lobes. These findings provide intriguing indirect support for the contention that lithium use increases neuronal viability/function in the human brain, and suggest that some of lithium's beneficial effects may be mediated by neurotrophic/neuroprotective events

It is hypothesized that lithium could act to prevent onset of psychosis in vulnerable young people through its neuroprotective effects as outlined above. Further, lithium is considered a well-tolerated medication with relatively few side-effects (Abou-Saleh and Coppen 1989; Dunner

2000)—two essential criteria for treatment for UHR young people. There is currently an open label trial, headed by Dr Gregor Berger and funded by the Stanley Foundation, using lithium in progress at the PACE Clinic.

Psychological treatments

As mentioned above, the first intervention trial in a UHR group included cognitive behavioural therapy in the treatment arm of the study (McGorry et al 2002). As this was combined with low dose risperidone it was difficult to elucidate which was the more active component of the intervention. Thus our subsequent study design has separated antipsychotic medication and cognitive therapy. This RCT is currently in progress.

The EDIE group has compared the impact of cognitive-behaviour oriented psychotherapy to monitoring alone (ie no psychological treatment) on the rate of transition to psychosis in 23 young people meeting UHR criteria. After 26 sessions of therapy only one of the 13 participants (8%) in this group had developed psychosis compared to four of the 11 in the monitoring group (36%) (French 2002; French et al 2003).

Conclusion

In conclusion, research in UHR individuals provides a unique opportunity to investigate the onset of psychotic disorder. The identification of people who are possibly incipient for psychosis allows exploration of the biological, psychological and social processes associated with this transition. This is of major importance for the future development of early intervention strategies. However, such research is dependent on our ability to accurately detect and predict which young people are truly at the highest risk. Hence, the ongoing evaluation of UHR criteria and identification of additional factors that make the development of psychosis even more likely are necessary. Exploration of other candidate risk factors, for example, cognitive abnormalities, eye movement disorders, further structural and functional brain abnormalities, and the role of stress and life events is needed. The influence of substance abuse requires further investigation. Family factors that may influence psychosis onset could also be studied. Further examination of which treatments might be most effective in this group is also crucial.

Along with these areas of study we must not lose sight of the ethical issues that such innovative work generates. Issues, such as stigma and labelling of non-psychotic people as 'prodromal for psychosis', the distribution of health resources and the use of antipsychotic medication in people without psychoses are some of these. We must ensure that methodologically sound research underpins any widespread shifts in practice or policy. Appropriate dissemination and discussion of results is also essential. The potential benefits to many young people and their families from this research are great.

Summary

- Research into the prodromal or pre-psychotic phase of schizophrenia and related disorders has been undertaken for around a decade with interesting results now emerging.
- The UHR criteria has now been validated in longitudinal studies in a number of sites around the world.
- Clinical variables that predict onset of psychosis over and above UHR criteria have

now been identified: belonging to both the Attenuated and Trait Groups, duration of symptoms greater than 5 years, low functioning according to the GAF and disorganization (according to the SANS). Together, these variables (in addition to meeting ARMS criteria) had a high specificity, positive predictive value and negative predictive value of transition to acute psychosis within 12 months.

- Results from neuroimaging studies suggest that there might be structural brain changes occurring around the time of transition to psychosis and that there are differences in brain structure prior to the transition to psychosis that differentiate between those ultra high risk (UHR) patients who will develop psychosis and those who will not.
- UHR individuals who later developed a schizophrenia spectrum disorder displayed a significant impairment in olfactory identification ability at baseline compared to UHR individuals who did not develop psychosis, UHR individuals who developed a non-schizophrenia spectrum disorder and a healthy comparison group. These findings could suggest that the incipient onset of schizophrenia compromises normal frontal lobe development and therefore interferes with the development of neuropsychological functions mediated by these regions.
- UHR patients perform intermediate to first episode psychosis and healthy control subjects on a range of neurocognitive tests. UHR patients who later developed psychosis performed worse on tests of logical memory, spatial working memory and information processing than UHR patients who did not.

- A range of other potential vulnerability markers for psychosis is being assessed in the UHR population including obstetric complications, childhood milestone achievement, substance abuse and membrane lipid biochemistry.
- Possible etiological factors for psychosis can be assessed in the UHR population. Studies are currently underway investigating the roles of viruses and HPA axis functioning in the onset of psychosis in the UHR population.
- Results of the first randomized control trials of antipsychotic medication and cognitive-behaviour therapy with UHR populations suggest that both interventions might have a role in treating the difficulties and problems UHR young people experience as well as delaying or preventing the onset of acute psychosis. There is scope for the investigation of a wide range of other approaches, including neuroprotective factors, such as lithium, in the treatment of the UHR population.

References

Abou-Saleh MT, Coppen A (1989) The efficacy of low-dose lithium: Clinical, psychological and biological correlates. *J Psychiatr Res* 23:157–162.

Alexander RC, Cabirac G, Lowenkopf T, et al (1992) Search for evidence of herpes simplex virus, type 1 or varicella-zoster virus infection in postmortem brain tissue from schizophrenic patients. *Acta Psychiatr Scand* 86:418–420.

Altamura C, Guercetti C, Percudani M (1989) Dexamethasone suppression test in positive and negative schizophrenia. *Psychiatry Res* 30:69–75.

American Psychiatric Association (1987) *DSM-III-R: Diagnostic and statistical manual for mental disorders* (3rd edn, rev). Washington DC: American Psychiatric Association.

American Psychiatric Association (1994) *DSM-IV: Diagnostic and statistical manual for mental disorders* (4th edn, rev). Washington DC: American Psychiatric Association.

Andreasen N (1982) Negative symptoms in schizophrenia: Definition and reality. *Arch Gen Psychiatry* 39:784–788.

Berger GE, Wood SJ, Pantelis C, et al (2002) Implications of lipid biology for the pathogenesis of schizophrenia. *Aust NZ J Psychiatry* 36:355–366.

Block W, Bayer TA, Tepest R, et al (2000) Decreased frontal lobe ratio of *N*-acetyl aspartate to choline in familial schizophrenia: a proton magnetic resonance spectroscopy study. *Neurosci Lett* 289:147–151.

Brewer WJ, Edwards J, Anderson V, et al (1996) Neuropsychological, olfactory, and hygiene deficits in men with negative symptom schizophrenia. *Biol Psychiatry* 40:1021–1031.

Brewer WJ, Francey SM, Wood SJ, et al (in prep) Cognition is impaired in patients at ultra high-risk for psychosis who later develop psychosis.

Brewer WJ, Pantelis C, Anderson V, et al (2001) Stability of olfactory identification deficits in neuroleptic-naive patients with first episode psychosis. *Am J Psychiatry* 158:107–115.

Brewer WJ, Wood SJ, McGorry PD, et al (2003) Olfactory identification ability is impaired in individuals at ultra high risk for psychosis who later develop schizophrenia. *Am J Psychiatry* 160: 1790–1794.

Brown AS, Cohen P, Greenwald S, Susser E (2000) Nonaffective psychosis after prenatal exposure to rubella. *Am J Psychiatry* 157:438–443.

Brown G, Birley J (1968) Crises and life changes and the onset of schizophrenia. *Health Soc Behav* 9:203–214.

Cadenhead K (2002) Vulnerability markers in the schizophrenia spectrum: Implications for phenomenology, genetics and the identification of the schizophrenia prodrome. *Psychiatr Clin North Am* 25:837–853.

Cannon TD, Mednick SA (1993) The schizophrenia high-risk project in Copenhagen: Three decades of progress. *Acta Psychiatr Scand* 87(suppl 370):33–47.

Cannon-Spoor HE, Potkin SG, Wyatt RJ (1982) Measurement of premorbid adjustment in chronic schizophrenia. *Schizophr Bull* **8**: 470–484.

Canton G, Fraccon IG (1985) Life events and schizophrenia: A replication. *Acta Psychiatr Scand* 71:211–216.

Carr V, Halpin S, Lau N, et al (2000) A risk factor screening and assessment protocol for schizophrenia and related psychosis. *Aust NZ J Psychiatry* 34(suppl):170–180.

Carter G I, Taylor GR, Crow TJ (1987) Search for viral nucleic acid sequences in the postmortem brains of patients with schizophrenia and individuals who have committed suicide. *J Neurol Neurosurg Psychiatry* 5:247–251.

Chung R K, Langeluddecke P, Tennant C (1986) Threatening life events in the onset of schizophrenia, schizophreniform psychosis and hypomania. *Br J Psychiatry* 148:680–685.

Clancy J, Crowe R, Winokur G, Morrison J (1973) The Iowa 500: Precipitating factors in schizophrenia and primary affective disorder. *Compr Psychiatry* 14:197–202.

Conejero-Goldberg C, Torrey EF, Yolken RH (2003) Herpesviruses and *Toxoplasma gondii* in orbital frontal cortex of psychiatric patients. *Schizophr Res* 60:65–69.

Cornblatt B A, Risch NJ, Faris G, et al (1988) The Continuous Performance Test, Identical Pairs version (CPT-IP): New findings about sustained attention in normal families. *Psychiatry Res* 26:223–238.

Cornblatt B, Lencz, T, Correll C, et al (2002a) Treating the prodrome: Naturalistic findings from the RAP Program. *Acta Psychiatr Scand Suppl* **106**: 44.

Cornblatt B, Lencz, T, Obuchowski MJ (2002b) The schizophrenia prodrome: Treatment and high-risk perspectives. *Schizophr Res* **54**:177–186.

Cotter DR, Pariante CM, Everall IP (2001) Glial cell abnormalities in major psychiatric disorders: the evidence and implications. *Brain Res Bull* 55:585–595.

Coyle JT, Schwarcz, R (2000) Mind glue: implications of glial cell biology for psychiatry. *Arch Gen Psychiatry* 57: 90–93.

de Lisi LE, Smith SB, Hamovit JR, et al (1986) Herpes simplex virus, cytomegalovirus and Epstein-Barr virus antibody titres in sera from schizophrenic patients. *Psychol Med* **16**:757–763.

Dunner DL (2000) Optimizing lithium treatment. *J Clin Psychiatry* **61**(suppl):76–81.

Eaton WW, Romanoski A, Anthony J C, Nestadt G (1991) Screening for psychosis in the general population with a self-report interview. *J Nerv Ment Dis* 179:689–693.

Erlenmeyer-Kimling L, Squires-Wheeler E, Adamo, UH, et al (1995) The New York High Risk Project: Psychoses and cluster A personality disorders in offspring of schizophrenic parents at 23 years of follow-up. *Arch Gen Psychiatry* 52:857–865.

Falloon IRH (1992) Early intervention for first episodes of schizophrenia: A preliminary exploration. *Psychiatry* **55**:4–15.

Falloon IR (2000) General practice recruitment for people at risk of schizophrenia: the Buckingham experience. *Aust NZ J Psychiatry;* 34(suppl):S131–S136.

Falloon IRH, Krekorian H, Shanahan WJ, et al (1990) The Buckingham project: A comprehensive mental health service based upon behavioural psychotherapy. *Behav Change* 7:51–57.

Francey SM (2002) *Predicting psychosis: A longitudinal investigation of prodromal features and neurocognitive vulnerability in young people at risk of psychosis.* Unpublished PhD thesis, University of Melbourne, NSW, Australia.

French P (2002) Model-driven psychological intervention to prevent onset of psychosis. *Acta Psychiatr Scand Suppl* **106**:18.

French P, Morrison AP, Walford L, et al (2003) Cognitive therapy for preventing transition to psychosis in high risk individuals: A case series. *Behav Cog Psychotherapy* **31**:53– 67.

Geddes JR, Lawrie SM (1995a) Obstetric complications and schizophrenia: A meta-analysis. *Br J Psychiatry* 167:786–793.

Geddes JR, Lawrie SM (1995b) Obstetric complications, neurodevelopmental deviance and risk of schizophrenia. *J Psychiatric Res* 21:413–421.

Gross G (1989) The 'basic' symptoms of schizophrenia. *Br J Psychiatry* **7**(suppl):21–5

Gruen R, Baron M (1984) Stressful life events and schizophrenia: Relation to illness onset and family history. *Neuropsychobiology* **12**:206–208.

Hall W, Hando, J (1994) Route of administration and adverse effects of amphetamine use in young adults in Sydney, Australia. *Drug Alcohol Rev* **13**:277–284.

Hambrecht M, Lammertink M, Klosterkötter J, et al (2002) Subjective and objective neuropsychological abnormalities in a psychosis prodrome clinic. *Br J Psychiatry* **181**(suppl):30–37.

Hamilton M (1960) A rating scale for depression. *J Neurol Neurosurg Pychiatry* **23**: 56–61.

Harrison PJ, Roberts GW (2000) *The neuropathology of schizophrenia.* Oxford University Press.

Hart DJ, Heath RG, Sautter FJ Jr, et al (1999) Antiretroviral antibodies: Implications for schizophrenia, schizophrenia spectrum disorders, and bipolar disorder. *Biol Psychiatry* **45**:704–714.

Hawkins KA, Addington J, Keefe RS, et al (2003) *Neuropsychological status of subjects putatively prodromal for a first episode of psychosis.* Paper presented at the International Congress on Schizophrenia Research, Colorado Springs, Colorado.

Heinrichs RW, Zakzanis KK (1998) Neurocognitive deficit in schizophrenia: A quantitative review of the evidence. *Neuropsychology* **12**:426–445.

Horrobin DF, Manku MS, Hillman H, et al (1991) Fatty acid levels in the brains of schizophrenics and normal controls. *Biol Psychiatry* **30**:795–805.

Hudson CJ, Lin A, Cogan S, et al (1997) The niacin challenge test: Clinical manifestation of altered transmembrane signal transduction in schizophrenia? *Biol Psychiatry* **41**:507–513.

Ingraham L J, Kugelmass S, Frenkel E, et al (1995) Twenty-five year follow-up of the Israeli High-risk Study: Current and lifetime psychopathology. *Schizophr Bull* **21**:183–192.

Jacobs S, Myers J (1976) Recent life events and acute schizophrenic psychosis: A controlled study. *J Nerv Ment Dis;* **162**: 75–87.

Jansen LMC, Gispen-de Wied CC, Kahn RS (1999) *Coping with Stress in Schizophrenia.* Presented at VIIth International Congress on Schizophrenia Research, Santa Fe, New Mexico.

Jarskog LF, Gilmore, JH, Selinger ES, Lieberman JA (2000) Cortical Bcl-2 protein expression and apoptotic regulation in schizophrenia. *Biol Psychiatry* **48**:641–650.

Kaneko M, Yokoyama F, Hoshino Y, et al (1992) Hypothalamic-pituitary-adrenal axis function in chronic schizophrenia: Association with clinical features. *Biol Psychiatry* **25**:1–7.

Karlsson H, Bachmann S, Schroder J, et al (2001) Retroviral RNA identified in the cerebrospinal fluids and brains of individuals with schizophrenia. *Proc Nat Acad Sci USA* **98**:4634–4639.

Kay SR, Fiszbein A, Opler LA (1987) The positive and negative syndrome scale (PANSS) for schizophrenia. *Schizophr Bull* **13**:261–269.

King M, Coker E, Leavey G, et al (1994) Incidence of psychotic illness in London: Comparison of ethnic groups. *BMJ* **309**:1115–1119.

Klosterkötter J (1992) The meaning of basic symptoms for the development of schizophrenic psychoses. *Neurol Psychiatry Brain Res* **1**:30–41.

Klosterkötter J, Ebel H, Schultze-Lutter F, Steinmeyer EM (1996) Diagnostic validity of basic symptoms. *Eur Arch Psychiatry Clin Neurosci* **246**:147–154.

Kovasznay B, Fleischer J, Tanenberg-Karant M, et al (1997) Substance use disorder and the early course of illness in schizophrenia and affective psychosis. *Schizophr Bull* **23**: 195–201.

Kremen WS, Seidman LJ, Pepple JR, et al (1994) Neuropsychological risk indicators for schizophrenia: a review of family studies. *Schizophr Bull* **20**:103–119.

Lammers CH, Garcia-Borreguero D, Schmider J, et al (1995) Combined dexamethasone/corticotropin-releasing hormone test in patients with schizophrenia and in normal controls: II. *Biol Psychiatry* **38**:803–807.

Larsen T K (2002) The transition from the premorbid period to psychosis: How can it be described? *Acta Psychiatr Scand Suppl* **106**:10–11.

Lencz, T, Smith CW, Auther A, et al (in press) The assessment of 'prodromal schizophrenia': Unresolved issues and future directions. *Schizophr Bull*

Lewis S, Murray R (1987) Obstetric complications, neurodevelopmental deviance, and the risk of schizophrenia. *J Psychiatr Res* **21**:413–421

Lin A, Kenis G, Bignotti S, et al (1988) The inflammatory response system in treatment-resistant schizophrenia: increased serum interleukin-6. *Schizophr Res* **32**:9–15.

Linszen DH, Dingemans PM Lenoir ME (1994) Cannabis abuse and the course of recent-onset schizophrenic disorders. *Arch Gen Psychiatry* **51**:273–279.

Malzacher M, Merz, J, Ebonther D (1981) Einscheidende Lebensereignisse im vorfeld akuter schizophrener Episoden. *Arch Psychiatrie Nervenkrank* **230**:227–242.

Manji HK, Moore GJ, Chen G (1999) Lithium at 50: Have the neuroprotective effects of this unique cation been overlooked? *Biol Psychiatry* **46**:929–940.

Manji HK, Moore GJ, Chen G (2000a) Lithium up-regulates the cytoprotective protein Bcl-2 in the CNS in vivo: A role for neurotrophic and neuroprotective effects in manic depressive illness. *J Clin Psychiatry* **61**(suppl 9):82–96.

Manji HK, Moore GJ, Chen G (2000b) Clinical and preclinical evidence for the neurotrophic effects of mood stabilizers: Implications for the pathophysiology and treatment of manic-depressive illness. *Biol Psychiatry* **48**:740–744.

Mazure CM, Quinlan DM, Bowers MB (1997) Recent life stressors and biological markers in newly admitted psychotic patients. *Biol Psychiatry* **41**:865–870.

McFarlane WR, Cook WL, Robbins D, Downing D (2002) Portland identification and early referral. *Acta Psychiatr Scand* **413**:20.

McGlashan TH, Zipursky RB, Perkins DO, et al (2002) *Olanzapine vs. placebo treatment of the schizophrenia prodrome: One-year results.* Paper presented at the ICOSR, Colorado Springs, Colorado.

McGlashan TH, Zipursky RB, Perkins D, et al (2003) The PRIME North America randomized double-blind clinical trial of olanzapine versus placebo in patients at risk of being prodromally symptomatic for psychosis: I. Study rationale and design. *Schizophr Res* **61**:7–18.

McGorry PD, Yung AR, Phillips LJ, et al (2002) Randomized controlled trial of interventions designed to reduce the risk of progression to first-episode psychosis in a clinical sample with subthreshold symptoms. *Arch Gen Psychiatr* **59**:921–928.

McNeil TF, Cantor-Graae E (2000) Minor physical anomalies and obstetric complications in schizophrenia. *Aust NZ J Psychiatry* **34**(suppl):S65–S73.

Meltzer HY, Lee MA, Jayathilake K (2001) The blunted plasma cortisol response to apomorphine and its relationship to treatment response in patients with schizophrenia. *Neuropsychopharmacology* **24**:278–290.

Miller TJ, McGlashan TH, Rosen JL, et al (2002) Prospective diagnosis of the initial prodrome for schizophrenia based on the Structured Interview for Prodromal Symptoms: Preliminary evidence of interrater and predictive validity. *Am J Psychiatry* **159**:863–865.

Miller TJ, Zipursky RB, Perkins D, et al (2003) The PRIME North America randomized double-blind clinical trial of olanzapine versus placebo in patients at risk of being prodromally symptomatic for psychosis: II. Baseline characteristics of the 'prodromal' sample. *Schizophr Res* **61**:19–30.

Miller T J, McGlashan TH, Rosen JL, et al (in press) Prodromal assessment with the Structured Interview for Prodromal Syndromes and the Scale of Prodromal Symptoms: Predictive validity, inter-rater reliability and training to reliability. *Schizophr Bull*

Miller W R, Rollnick S (1991) *Motivational interviewing: Preparing people to change addictive behaviour.* New York: Guildford Press.

Moberg PJ, Doty RL, Turetsky BI, et al (1997) Olfactory identification deficits in schizophrenia - correlation with duration of illness. *Am J Psychiatry* **154**:1016–1018.

Mojabai R, Malaspina D, Susser E (in press) The promise of primary prevention in schizophrenia: Concepts and assumptions. *Schizophr Bull*

Moore GJ, Bebchuk JM, Hasanat K, et al (2000) Lithium increases *N*-acetyl-aspartate in the human brain: in vivo evidence in support of bcl-2's neurotrophic effects? *Biol Psychiatry* **48**:1–8.

Morrison AP, Bentall RP, French P, et al (2002) Randomised controlled trial of early detection and cognitive therapy for preventing transition to psychosis in high-risk individuals. Study design and interim analysis of transition rate and psychological risk factors. *Br J Psychiatry* **43**(suppl):S78–S84.

Mück-Seler D, Pivac N, Jakovljevic M, Brzovic Z (1999) Platelet serotonin, plasma cortisol and dexamethasone suppression test in schizophrenic patients. *Biol Psychiatry* **45**:1433–1439.

Müller N, Riedel M, Ackenheil M, Schwarz, MJ (1999) The role of immune function in schizophrenia: an overview. *Eur Arch Psychiatry Clin Neurosci* **249**:62–68.

Murray R, Lewis SW (1987) Is schizophrenia a neurodevelopmental disorder? *Br Med J* **295**:681–682.

Nikkila HV, Muller K, Ahokas A, et al (1999) Accumulation of macrophages in the CSF of schizophrenic patients during acute psychotic episodes. *Am J Psychiatry* **156**:1725–1729.

O'Brien JT (1997) The 'glucocorticoid cascade' hypothesis in man. *Br J Psychiatry* **170**:199–201.

O'Reilly RL (1994) Viruses and schizophrenia. *Aust NZ J Psychiatry* **28**:222–228.

Pantelis C, Yücel M, Wood SJ, et al (2003a) Early and late neurodevelopmental disturbances in schizophrenia and their functional consequences. *Aust NZ J Psychiatry* **37**:399–406.

Pantelis C, Velakoulis D, McGorry PD, et al (2003b) Neuroanatomical abnormalities before and after onset of psychosis: A cross-sectional and longitudinal MRI study. *Lancet* **361**:281–288.

Peters E, Day S, McKenna J, Orbach G (1999a) Delusional ideation in religious and psychotic populations. *Br J Clin Psychol* **38**:83–96.

Peters ER, Joseph SA, Garety PA (1999b) Measurement of delusional ideation in the normal population: Introducing the PDI [Peters et al Delusions Inventory]. *Schizophr Bull* **25**: 553–576.

Phillips LJ, Curry C, Yung AR, et al (2002a) Cannabis use is not associated with the development of psychosis in an 'ultra' high-risk group. *Aust NZ J Psychiatry* **36**:800–806.

Phillips LJ, Velakoulis D, Pantelis C, et al (2002b) Non-reduction in hippocampal volume is associated with higher risk of psychosis. *Schizophr Res* **58**:145–158.

Rabinowitz, J, Bromet EJ, Lavelle J, et al (1998) Prevalence and severity of substance use disorders and onset of psychosis in first-admission psychotic patients. *Psychol Med* **28**:411–419.

Rapaport MH, Lohr JB (1994) Serum-soluble interleukin-2 receptors in neuroleptic-naive schizophrenic subjects and in medicated schizophrenic subjects with and without tardive dyskinesia. *Acta Psychiatr Scand* **90**:311–315.

Sapolsky RM, Romero, LM, Munck AU (2000) How do glucocorticoids influence stress responses? Integrating permissive, suppressive, stimulatory and preparative actions. *Endocr Rev* **21**:55–89.

Satel SL, Southwick SM, Gawin FH (1991) Clinical features of cocaine induced paranoia. *Am J Psychiatr* **148**:495–498.

Schwartz, CC, Myers JK (1977) Life events and schizophrenia:II. Impact of life events on symptom configuration. *Arch Gen Psychiatry* **34**:1242–1245.

Schwarz, MJ, Ackenheil M, Riedel M, Muller N (1998) Blood-cerebrospinal fluid barrier impairment as indicator for an immune process in schizophrenia. *Neurosci Lett* **253**:201–203.

Seidman LJ, Goldstein JM, Goodman JM, et al (1997) Sex differences in olfactory identification and Wisconsin card sorting performance in schizophrenia: Relationship to attention and verbal ability. *Biol Psychiatry* **42**:104–115.

Shah SH, Vankar GK, Peet M, Ramchand CN (2000) Unmedicated schizophrenic patients have a reduced skin flush in response to topical niacin. *Schizophr Res* **43**:163–164.

Shenton ME, Dickey CC, Frumin M, McCarley RW (2001) A review of MRI findings in schizophrenia. *Schizophr Res* **49**:1–52.

Srikanth S, Ravi V, Poornnima KS, et al (1994) Viral antibodies in recent onset, nonorganic psychoses: Correspondence with symptomatic severity. *Biol Psychiatry* **36**:517–521.

Steele TD, McCann UD, Ricaurte GA (1994) 3,4-Methylenedioxymethamphetamine (MDMA), 'ecstasy': Pharmacology and toxicology in animals and humans. *Addiction* 89:539–545.

Strassman RJ (1984) Adverse reactions to psychedelic drugs: A review of the literature. *J Nerv Ment Dis* 172:577–582.

Tart C (1970) Marijuana intoxication: Common experiences. *Nature* 226:701–704.

Thomas H (1993) Psychiatric symptoms in cannabis users. *Br J Psychiatry;*163:141–149.

Tien A, Anthony J (1990) Epidemiological analysis of alcohol and drug use as risk factors for psychotic experiences. *J Nerv Ment Dis* 178:473–480.

Torrey E F (1988) Stalking the schizovirus. *Schizophr Bull* 14:223–229.

van den Bosch RJ, van Asma MJO, Rambouts R, Louwerens JW (1992) Coping style and cognitive dysfunction in schizophrenic patients. *Br J Psychiat* 161: 123–128.

van Os J, Hanssen M, Bijl R V, Ravelli A (2000) Strauss (1969) revisited: A psychosis continuum in the general population? *Schizophr Res* 45:11–20.

van Os J, Hanssen M, Bijl R V, Vollebergh W (2001) Prevalence of psychotic disorder and community level of psychotic symptoms: an urban-rural comparison. *Arch Gen Psychiatry* 58:663–668.

Vance AL, Velakoulis D, Maruff P, et al (1999) Magnetic resonance spectroscopy and schizophrenia: What have we learnt? *Aust NZ J Psychiatry* 34:14–25.

Velakoulis D, Pantelis C, McGorry PD, et al (1999) Hippocampal volume in first-episode psychoses and chronic schizophrenia: A high resolution Magnetic Resonance Imaging study. *Arch Gen Psychiatry* 56:33–40.

Ward LC (1990) Prediction of verbal, performance and full scale IQs from seven subtests of the WAIS-R. *J Clin Psychol* 46:436–440.

Ward PE, Sutherland J, Glen EM, Glen AI (1998) Niacin skin flush in schizophrenia: A preliminary report. *Schizophr Res* 29:269–274.

Wechsler D (1981) *Weschler adult intelligence scale – Revised (Manual).* New York: The Psychological Corporation

Weinberger DE (1987) Implications of normal brain development for the pathogenesis of schizophrenia. *Arch Gen Psychiatry* 44:660–669.

Weinberger DR (1999) Cell biology of the hippocampal formation in schizophrenia. *Biol Psychiatry* 45:395–402.

Wolf LE, Cornblatt BA (1996) Neuropsychological functioning in children at risk for schizophrenia. In Pantelis C, Nelson HE, Barnes TRE, eds, *Schizophrenia: A neuropsychological perspective.* Chichester, UK: Wiley.

Wood SJ, Berger G, Velakoulis D, et al (in press) Proton magnetic resonance spectroscopy in first episode and ultra high-risk individuals. *Schizophr Bull*

Wood SJ, Pantelis C, Proffitt T, et al (2003) Spatial working memory ability is a marker of risk-for-psychosis. *Psychol Med* 33: 1239–1247.

Woods SW, Breier A, Zipursky RB, et al (in press) Randomized trial of olanzapine vs placebo in the symptomatic acute treatment of the schizophrenic prodrome. *Biol Psychiatry.*

Yao JK, Leonard S, Reddy RD (2000) Membrane phospholipid abnormalities in postmortem brains from schizophrenic patients. *Schizophr Res* 42:7–17.

Yehuda R, Southwick SM, Nussbaum G, et al (1990) Low urinary cortisol excretion in patients with posttraumatic stress disorder. *J Nerv Ment Dis* 178:366–369.

Yehuda R, Boisoneau D, Mason JW et al (1993) Glucocorticoid receptor number and cortisol secretion in mood, anxiety and psychotic disorders. *Biol Psychiatry* 34:18–25.

Yeragani VK (1990) The incidence of abnormal dexamethasone suppression in schizophrenia: A review and a meta-analytic comparison with the incidence in normal controls. *Can J Psychiatry* 35:128–132.

Yolken RH, Torrey EF (1995) Viruses, schizophrenia and bipolar disorder. *Clin Microbiol Rev* 8:131–145.

Yücel M, Wood SJ, Phillips LJ, et al (2003) Morphology of the anterior cingulate cortex in young men at ultra high risk of developing a psychotic illness. *Br J Psychiatry* 182:518–524.

Yung AR, Phillips LJ, McGorry PD, et al (1998) Can we predict onset of first episode psychosis in a high risk group? *Int Clin Psychopharmacol* **13**(suppl 1):S23–S30.

Yung AR, Phillips LJ, Yuen HP, et al (2003) Psychosis prediction: 12 month follow-up of a high risk ('prodromal') group. *Schizophr Res* **60**:21–32.

Yung AR, Phillips LJ, Yuen HP, McGorry PD (in press) Risk factors for psychosis: Psychopathology and clinical features. *Schizophr Res.*

Future directions

8

The ultimate goal of better characterization of the onset of psychotic disorders including schizophrenia is prevention of the full expression of the disorder and hence the reduction of incidence, prevalence and associated morbidity and mortality. This chapter will describe the context for preventive strategies for mental disorders in young people, and characterize the challenges and opportunities that exist in this crucial arena of public health. First, we consider the mental health of young people in general, consider the fundamental question of how to define a mental disorder, and then focus on the best mix of preventive strategies. Finally, we outline the kind of studies, models and treatments that need to be developed to underpin further progress.

The rising tide of mental disorders in young people

In recent years, the developed world has become increasingly conscious of one of major paradoxes of modern society. As the physical and material health and well-being of young people in developed countries has progressively improved during the second half of the 20th century, there has been a steady and alarming decline in their mental health. The period between 12 and 26 years has always been the phase of life during which severe psychiatric disorder is at its peak. However there is now solid scientific evidence that the prevalence and complexity of disorders have increased (Rutter and Smith 1995). This means that the core mental disorders, together with a confusing comorbid admixture of emotional distress and problem behaviours, are more common than ever before. For example, more than one in four (27%) 18 to 24-year-olds in the 1998 Australian National Survey of Mental Health and Well-being (Andrews et al 1999) had a diagnosable mental disorder.

The more dramatic manifestations of this 'rising tide', such as suicide, death from drug overdose and violent behaviour are featured daily in the media. Less dramatic are the erosive effects on the prospects and quality of life of these young people and their families, especially those who develop the core psychiatric illnesses during this phase of life, such as schizophrenia and bipolar disorder, and severe depression. Governments are well aware of this serious public health problem, but the response to date has been fragmentary and manifestly ineffective. A vital missing ingredient has been a cohesive and practical research strategy, which focuses on young adults as well as adolescents. It is our contention that if schizophrenia and related psychotic disorders are going to be detected and treated at the very early prodromal phase, then this is best done as part of a broader strategy focusing on the broad array of emerging mental disorders in this phase of life.

Epidemiology of serious mental illness and transition to adulthood: a negative synergy

This public health crisis represents the adding of fuel to a longstanding fire. Recent landmark surveys have revealed that the major psychiatric disorders, such as schizophrenia, bipolar disorder, depression and anxiety, substance abuse disorders, eating disorders and personality disorders, for the most part emerge for the first time in adolescence or young adult life, between the ages of 12 and 26 (Mrazek and Haggerty 1994). Large Australian surveys have confirmed

these findings and have found that the peak period for mental disorder is the young adult period between 18 and 24 years, where the rate of disorder of 27% is nearly double the 14% seen in children and younger adolescents (Andrews et al 1999; Sawyer et al 2000). However, mental health services for older adolescents and young adults are at best embryonic and poorly accessible, at worst non-existent. This pattern of peak onset in young people has probably always existed, for example, the original term for schizophrenia was 'dementia praecox'. However, the age of onset for some disorders, notably depression, appears to be getting earlier, hence the term 'downward developmental trend' (Zubrick et al 2000). Youth is not only the peak period for the onset of psychiatric symptoms, it is also a period in which major physical, hormonal and brain changes occur, and is a complex and often precarious phase in the life cycle for psychosocial development. There are many tasks to be accomplished, particularly the achievement of a secure sense of self, separation from the family, and the building of friendships, intimacy and a career (Aggleton et al 2000). These tasks have become much more complex and stressful, and frequently trigger mental disorders (Booth et al 1999). Conversely, mental disorders can seriously impede a young person's growth and development (Kessler et al 1995). They sap confidence and create unwanted dependence on parents just when autonomy should be increasing. Furthermore, young people typically do not know how to seek help for mental disorders, are reluctant to do so, and often fail to gain access, are frequently misunderstood or poorly treated when they do (Lincoln and McGorry 1999).

The original World Bank report on the global burden of disease (Murray and Lopez 1996) also highlighted that society has invested heavily in young people by early adulthood and the onset of death or disability at this phase of life represents a human and economic disaster. Mental and substance abuse disorders represent over two thirds of this burden of disease in the 15–24 year age group. Interestingly, the death or disability of young people in early adult life is also valued most highly in economic as well as human terms by these studies. The combination of the peak incidence of disorder in this age group, the high value placed on the health of young people, and the lack of any substantial mental health response, let alone a pro-active or early intervention focus provides a potent rationale and opportunity for major investment in research and development.

What is a disorder anyway?

Mrazek and Haggerty (1994) in their landmark report for the US Institute of Medicine on Prevention in Mental Disorders emphasize the need for research to map the prodromal and onset periods of potentially serious mental disorders and look for malleable risk and protective factors influencing progression of disorder. First episodes of illness however, especially in primary care settings, bear much less resemblance to prototypical diagnostic categories (eg schizophrenia), than the more established cases which are seen in tertiary settings. They are characterized especially in young people by striking and dynamically fluctuating levels of comorbidity. This makes the categorical definition of individual disorders or diagnoses difficult. We will probably need to work in a dimensional as well as a categorical framework with different thresholds of severity (McGorry et al 1995, 1998; Rutter 1998). This syndromal

diffusion is even more significant when subthreshold syndromes become the focus, as with the attempt to define and intervene during the prodromal phase in psychotic disorder. This difficulty was expanded upon in Chapter 3.

We need to consider what is a 'case' (Wing et al 1974) for two fundamental reasons. The first is to judge whether treatment of some kind should be offered, and second to provide a framework for exploring the underlying causes of disorder.

> *People have problems before they have diagnoses.*
> Shiers D (Personal Communication,
> September 2002)

> *Classification is a simple—but fundamental— step that is mandatory if we are to understand psychopathology. Classification is a basic human process that we all use to understand our environment. In the mental health field, we need a classification of psychopathology in order to help us understand what we clinicians deal with—people who have problems in living.*
> Blashfield (1984: viii–ix)

Blashfield also describes psychopathology from the perspective of the patient as an 'unmarked sea' for which there exist no maps or charts. This was also true for the clinician during the 19th century when no clear boundaries were obvious within the vast array of symptoms present in their patients. Since then, artificial boundaries based on syndromal clusters, often confounded (eg in the case of schizophrenia) with prognostic or course variables, have been established. Given the lack of progress in clarifying specific underlying pathophysiology, this is an unsatisfactory situation, and consequently psychiatric diagnosis has been a shaky enterprise for much of this century. Serious questioning of the reliability and validity of psychiatric diagnosis in the 1960s and 1970s ushered in the current era of operationally defined diagnoses, underpinned by diagnostic manuals, notably DSM-III (American Psychiatric Association, 1980) and its successors, and ICD-10 (World Health Organization, 1992). While a temporary improvement, these reforms have not solved the problem of validity and have created a spurious precision (McGorry et al 1989, 1995). Defining the boundary between normality on the one hand, and between individual disorders, on the other remains a challenge. This challenge is greatly magnified in relation to the initial onset of disorder as highlighted in Chapter 3.

As in other branches of medicine, diagnostic concepts derived in tertiary settings, have proved to have much less applicability in other clinical settings. For example, the DSM categories for anxiety and depressive disorders mesh poorly with the comorbid pictures seen in primary care and community surveys (Goldberg and Huxley 1992). For similar reasons, diagnostic concepts derived from subsamples of patients with chronic disease, especially when the criteria require a certain duration or course, as in schizophrenia and bipolar disorder, do not work well in the early or onset phases of disorder. Here, there is much greater variability of psychiatric symptoms, more comorbidity, more syndromal flux, and more 'misdiagnosis' according to later diagnoses based on a more 'chronic' diagnostic model (Carlson et al 1994; Fennig et al 1994; Joyce 1984; McGorry et al 1990). The clinician's experience in this phase, especially in more primary settings, is that the diagnostic models are unwieldy and do not fit the clinical reality. The concept of 'goodness of fit', based on a prototypical model of diagnosis, utilized in ICD-10 diagnostic field trials could be helpful here.

Trying to apply the traditional diagnostic models frequently leads to confusion regarding what to treat and when.

Our group has looked at this issue within psychotic disorders and in common with other researchers (van Os et al 1999a and b) found tremendous variability, overlap and dimensionality in the psychopathology of broadly defined first episode psychosis patients (Bell et al 1998; McGorry 1991; McGorry et al 1998; van Os et al 1996). In the prepsychotic phase (Häfner et al 1995; McGorry et al 1995; Yung and McGorry 1996a; Yung et al 2003), even greater diversity of symptoms both cross-sectionally and longitudinally has been found. The task of predicting subsequent, more dominant or severe, syndromes, even broad ones like 'psychosis', is a real challenge (Yung et al 2003). Predicting stable schizophrenia or bipolar disorder from subthreshold features, even more so. In young people more broadly, the constant clinical task is to distinguish between those who have problems in living, which are self-limited and within the normal range, and those who have a true mental disorder. Here again, the ubiquity of comorbidity seems to undermine the utility of a disorder-based approach. Yet, dimensional systems in which each aspect or problem is graded by severity are unwieldy or unworkable.

The recent surveys which demonstrate high levels of morbidity in the general population (Andrews et al 1999) have also raised the question of what actually constitutes a disorder, and especially a disorder that needs treatment (Andrews 1999; Regier et al 1998). It has also been belatedly pointed out that whatever these surveys are measuring, they are not accurately defining clinically significant disorder (Frances 1998). One obvious approach is to link the threshold for caseness to impact of the disorder in terms of burden or disability (Regier et al 1998). When this was done in the young adult population in the Netherlands, the prevalence of DSM-III-R psychiatric disorder in young adults aged between 19 and 24 years was reduced from 19% to 14% (moderate disability) and to 5% (severe disability) (Ferdinand et al 1995). However, this is a cross-sectional strategy, which immediately reduces the potential for early intervention or secondary prevention early in the course of disorder to limit such impact and disability. Requiring severe impact and disability to be already present is a hallmark of psychiatric care since services usually require frankly psychotic patients to demonstrate chronicity, suicidality or aggression, before responding or permitting access to and tenure within services. Finally, if such a disorder is present, is there effective treatment (a) in existence and (b) readily available and *deliverable* in the real world. The lack of confidence on the latter front has perhaps been an obstacle for developed countries, in particular, in implementing the logic of the World Bank Global Burden of Disease report (Murray and Lopez 1996). Is widespread deployment of existing psychiatric expertise possible and would it be cost effective in reducing the burden of disease?

Eaton (2001) has written most clearly about incidence and the issue of defining onset. He also contributed key concepts to the Institute of Medicine (US) report on prevention, which reformed the conceptual framework for prevention in mental health (Mrazek and Haggerty 1994). He points out that specific mental disorders are difficult to distinguish from non-morbid states, since symptoms taken alone are common. As discussed in Chapter 3, this is as true of psychotic symptoms as non-psychotic symptoms. The former have recently been shown

to occur commonly as isolated phenomena with no clear clinical significance (van Os et al 1999b, 2001). Young people especially seem to manifest the highest rates of these psychotic-like features (Verdoux et al 1998). Clustering of symptoms, especially the requirement that they cluster within a limited time-frame, has been used in operational criteria for disorders and is used to create the diagnostic concept. However, it is not well established that these clusters correspond well to other characteristics of disease entities, such as course, treatment response, and biological correlates. Hence, the lack of established validity of the criteria-based classification systems exacerbates problems of dating of the onset of disorder. This should make us cautious about conceptualizing the process of disease onset.

One criterion of onset in some studies is entry to treatment. This is inappropriate in psychiatry since so many people with mental disorders do not seek or obtain treatment for them. This is also true of even severe mental disorders, such as psychoses, even in developed countries and certainly in developing countries (Padmavathi et al 1998). Another criterion of onset is detectability—that is, when symptoms first appear. This is also unacceptable because experiences analogous to the symptoms of most psychiatric disorders are so widespread. We saw this in our survey of prodromal symptoms of schizophrenia in high school adolescents. While only a fraction of 1% could possibly have been truly prodromal (Jablensky 1999), at least 10–15% of the students reported two or more of these features persisting for significant periods (McGorry et al 1995). This is clearly true of other symptomatology, such as depression, though such symptoms do increase the risk of subsequent more severe disorder (Eaton 1995; Mrazek and Haggerty 1994).

Eaton (1995) feels it is preferable to conceptualize onset as a continuous line of development toward manifestation of a disease. There may be a threshold at which the development becomes irreversible, so that at some minimal level of symptomatology, it is certain that the full characteristics of the disease, however defined, will become apparent. Prior to this point, the symptoms are thought of as 'subcriterial' or subthreshold. Here, they can be seen as operating as a risk factor for the 'criterial' or full-threshold disorder. Intervention at this point falls into the indicated prevention category. Eaton argues that longitudinal studies are required to determine the levels of symptomatology at which irreversibility is achieved. This model is potentially useful but can be questioned in a number of ways. First, it may be that there is no point of irreversibility, and that disorders can recede at any time from the (arbitrary) threshold for criterial diagnosis. Second, and more fundamentally, the criterion or threshold in practice looks very much like an artefact. In the PACE Clinic, those patients who make the 'transition' to psychosis are not dramatically different before and after, the change is more a linear progression of severity than a 'psychotic break'. Similarly, psychotic relapse often looks more 'acute' in established disorder because of delayed treatment response, which only occurs after a behavioural incident. Finally, once the point of irreversibility, if there is one, is reached, this actually should become the operational definition of the threshold for the particular disorder.

Eaton's ideas about the development toward disease are also helpful. He argues that there are two perspectives or processes. The first is *intensification* of symptoms. These may have been present in a mild form for a long time, and

may never have been absent (such as personality traits). Here, the researcher must consider whether there is a crucial level of intensity of a given symptom or symptoms for which the rate of development toward a full-blown disease state is accelerated or becomes irreversible (see Case Study 2, Chapter 3). The second is the emergence of new symptoms that did not exist before. This involves the gradual *acquisition* of symptoms so that clusters are formed that increasingly approach the constellation required to meet specified definitions for diagnosis. When symptoms cluster or cohere in this way, more than expected by chance, they are regarded as forming a syndrome, which may be severe or non-severe. Hence, the symptom intensification process complements the idea of acquisition. The latter requires the researcher to consider the order in which symptoms occur over the natural history of disease and, in particular, whether one symptom is more important than another in accelerating the process. Receiver Operated Characteristics (ROC) analysis is a technique suited to exploring these relationships, provided the right data are available (Kraemer et al 2000; McGorry et al 2000).

Eaton defines incidence as the *force of morbidity* in the population, and acquisition and intensification as indicators of this. They are not tied to any particular threshold of caseness, which can be seen to be an arbitrary decision. In psychosis, we have tried to link case definition to the threshold for initiation of a particular treatment, that is, antipsychotic medication, rather than any current diagnostic manual's definition. Hence, we regard a week of severe and sustained delusions or hallucinations as marking the threshold for caseness (see Chapter 3 for criteria for identifying onset of psychosis). A treatment-oriented threshold for caseness could be set for all major syndromes, and could even vary depending on the individual treatment in question. For example, the threshold for counselling in depression may be lower than for drug therapy. This could be important because some disorders with high thresholds eg post-traumatic stress disorder or PTSD, panic disorder and major depression, many subthreshold cases are clearly distressed and disabled (Olfson et al 1996) yet may be wrongly excluded as 'met un-need' (Andrews and Henderson 2000). A different threshold and boundary may be appropriate when studying the underlying pathophysiology of psychiatric disorder.

This level of epidemiological sophistication has not yet been brought to bear on the onset phase of psychiatric disorders. The key objectives and preferred designs are highlighted in Mrazek and Haggerty (1994: 117–118). There is a strong preference for prospective designs, which have the potential to examine not only prodromal phases and precursor features as they wax, wane and cohere within and across putative syndromes, but also risk and protective factors for progression or remission. Such risk and protective factors are likely to be generic across a number of syndromes, although there may be higher valences for some syndromes than others, and the valences or potencies may change according to different phases of disorder and different developmental stages of the life cycle. Retrospective studies may still be useful in laying foundations for such prospective studies. We utilized this approach in reconstructing the psychotic prodrome (Yung and McGorry 1996b), as did Häfner and colleagues (Häfner et al 1995), before moving to a prospective model of research. This could be carried out for a range of disorders from substance abuse through bipolar disorder, major depression and anxiety

disorders. To do this, in the face of ubiquitous comorbidity, we need to invoke the concept of the *dominant* syndrome.

The dominant syndrome notion derives from hierarchical methods of psychiatric diagnosis (Boyd et al 1984). Here, one syndrome (eg Schneiderian or 'first rank' schizophrenia symptoms) is allowed to 'trump' all others, as in 'a trace of schizophrenia *is* schizophrenia', usually on theoretical grounds of dubious validity. An alternative is to pick the most severe, pervasive and persistent cluster of symptoms (eg a group of negative symptoms), and regard this as the dominant syndrome. If this is done we can select a subsample, according to the dominant syndrome, from within a larger group of first episode psychiatric patients with a severe disorder, and trace back retrospectively the prodromal and pretreatment course. We can map the waxing and waning of clinical features, complications and comorbid syndromes. Contrasting the onset phases of different subsamples would give a reasonable picture of the commonalities and differences between these, as well as points of divergence, when or if one syndrome became more stable and dominant. The main problem is that the concept and method of selection of the dominant syndromes may be flawed, though this still seems a reasonable way to start. Another variant is the prototype model of diagnosis, where the dominant syndrome could be selected via 'goodness of fit' to a predefined 'ideal type'.

A complementary and probably more productive strategy, although more complex, prolonged and expensive, would be to identify large samples of young people in the general population and follow them up from before puberty in a series of waves over a period of 10 years or longer. This has been done in a broad way by epidemiological researchers (eg Patton et al 2002). However, their focus has been mainly concerned with etiological risk factors than characterization of onset. A more focused initial strategy would be to identify a cohort of young people with a broad range of subthreshold symptoms and follow them up, perhaps over a shorter time-frame, and within this sampling frame conduct nested intervention studies (Cuijpers 2003). Flexible service structures to support these designs would need to be established. For example the PACE clinic concept (currently linked to ultra high risk for psychosis) could be broadened to the full range of subthreshold youth mental health problems. Initial broad spectrum interventions could be offered to all subthreshold subjects who would only need to meet an omnibus definition for 'at risk mental state', while studies examining more refined preventive interventions to reduce the risk of transition to particular 'dominant syndromes' could then be developed and offered at a secondary stage to subsets of patients or subjects meeting specific operational criteria. This would have the advantage of reducing stigma, bypassing and even exploiting the comorbidity issue more effectively, and improving recruitment, which has been an obstacle for pre-psychotic research.

A complementary research focus, which needs to be built into this stream of research, is the qualitative and ethnographic description of pathways to care and the topography and experience of help-seeking. This has been begun for young people with psychosis (Lincoln and McGorry 1999) and for adults with non-psychotic disorder, however these studies are very new in youth mental health (Biro et al 2002; Keys Young 1997).

Indicated prevention: the leading edge for prevention of mental disorders?

Probably the most important research goal in prevention research is determining which prevention strategies have the best chance of reducing the incidence of new cases of mental disorder. Cuijpers (2003) recently illustrated convincingly that at least for the purposes of research, indicated prevention is the most feasible of the preventive models for realistic reduction in incidence in both high and low incidence disorders.

Until recently, influenced by the views of Rose (1992), the most attractive preventive strategy for reducing incidence has been a universal or whole population approach. From a research perspective, for mental disorders the fundamental obstacle to examining the impact of universal and to a lesser extent selective prevention programmes is clearly the lack of statistical power. This in turn is related to the very low specificity of most known risk factors and the lack of understanding of the exact causal pathways leading to mental disorders. For example, for low incidence disorders, such as anorexia nervosa, millions of subjects would be required in a universal intervention programme to demonstrate a reduction in incidence of one third. For high incidence disorders, such as depression, the sample size required still runs to tens of thousands. Such studies are almost impossible to carry out because of the sheer numbers required. We therefore have little idea of what interventions might be effective, and furthermore there are other cost and ethical problems with such research. Selective interventions are also limited by power problems. The origins once again derive from the low specificity and lack of detailed knowledge regarding risk factors and their causal sequence and salience. Selective prevention may be feasible in some situations, however, the numbers required to examine the impact are likely to reach many hundreds in each intervention group. In stark contrast, indicated prevention, as predicted by Mrazek and Haggerty (1994) shapes as a much better bet. The sample sizes required for both high and low incidence disorders are much lower (approx 35–150) and this feasibility allows interventions to be developed and tested for their efficacy. The power for the low incidence disorders can be enhanced by two stage enrichment designs as in our own work. While this argument is presented from a prevention research perspective, it ultimately should hold for the public health task of reducing the incidence of disorder in the most cost-effective manner, at least until more is known about the causal pathways involving the multiple risk factors. Cuijpers (2003) goes on to list several ways to

increase the statistical power in prevention studies to which other strategies can be added (Table 8.1).

This analysis is instructive and more or less validates the approach taken so far in constructing the methodology for pre-psychotic research. It also shows how the paradigm can be extended to the full range of disorders in young people, suggesting mutual advantages for the reduction in incidence and prevalence of both high and low prevalence disorders, and how the universal, selective and indicated prevention strategies might be synergistically combined, cohering around the core of indicated prevention. So universal mental health promotion strategies might be combined with screening for asymptomatic and symptomatic (subthreshold) high risk groups for whom multimodal yet generic psychosocial interventions, (eg simple forms of cognitive-behaviour therapy or cognitive-analytic therapy) (Ryle 1995), could be offered aiming to reduce

Table 8.1
Strategies to increase statistical power in preventive studies (adapted from Cuijpers 2003)

A. Focus on and create populations with high incidence rates of mental disorder
- Focus on indicated prevention.
- Focus on high risk groups with multiple risk factors.
- Focus on target groups with multiple disorders.
- Develop multilevel screens to enrich for specific low incidence subsets within high incidence or broad spectrum samples.

B. Strengthen the effects of prevention programmes
- Need to target causal risk factors if known.
- Combine universal, selective and indicated paradigms.

C. Use cumulative meta-analyses
- Need multiple high quality comparable studies.

D. Use other methods
- Extend follow-up times.
- Use survival methods rather than fixed incidence counts.
- Improve the reliability of diagnoses.

the risk of multiple disorders. Follow-up arms could reveal those subjects whose symptoms continued or worsened and they could be subdivided according to second stage criteria and entered in studies to test more specific forms of indicated prevention targeting specific syndromal outcomes such as psychosis.

Future research designs

Some possible research design would be as follows:

- A series of retrospective reconstructions of the onset phase of several paradigmatic dominant syndromes (eg bipolar disorder, anorexia nervosa, substance abuse, severe depression, PTSD, panic disorder and obsessive-compulsive disorder). These would be done in relatively small samples ($n =$ 30–50) and include qualitative as well as quantitative approaches and depiction of the topography of pathways to care. Methodology would be based on the approaches used in the work of Yung (Yung and McGorry 1996b) and Lincoln (Lincoln and McGorry 1999).
- The assembly of a cohort with the full range of subthreshold symptomatology and follow-up of this sample over a medium term period (2–5 years). This may be linked with an appropriate clinical intervention examined within a randomized controlled trial (RCT) design.
- A community survey of psychiatric morbidity in young people aged between 15 and 24 years by expert (research psychologists) diagnostic interviewers to depict the boundaries of all syndromes with normal experience. This could form the foundation for a longitudinal study in stage 2 which could examine the dynamic

flux in symptoms over time and explore the models proposed by Eaton (2001) as well as other possibilities. It would also look at risk and protective factors for onset of disorder, such as stress, drug use, coping and social support, as well as experiences of help-seeking and the topography and response of the pathways to care.

Neurobiology and neuroprotection

Prospective research designs of this type also lend themselves to the intensive study of subsamples of subjects who meet ultra high risk criteria for progression or transition to a more stable dominant syndromal diagnosis. Increasing sophistication of neuroimaging paradigms and the capacity to map gene expression using genomic technology mean that it is possible to develop better understanding not only of the neurophysiological and neurochemical mechanisms involved in the onset and expression of psychiatric disorder, but also to select and evaluate the effectiveness of a new wave of agents that may be more directly neuroprotective of the developing and incipiently dysfunctional brain. Such agents may well be more subtle and benign in their effects. This neurobiological stream of research and therapeutics is highly compatible with increasing the sophistication of psychosocial interventions.

Conclusion

The development of the 'close-in' or ultra high risk (UHR) strategy in psychotic disorder represents a practical demonstration of indicated prevention in the real world. While there have been critics of this approach (Warner 2001), it is receiving increasing support from mainstream prevention researchers (Cuijpers 2003; Mrazek and Haggerty 1994) as being the most feasible current strategy in the prevention of mental disorders. Debate focuses on other related issues, notably ethical considerations, generalizability, and most importantly, what are the effective and safe interventions to be studied. This is a rich field for future etiological, clinical and epidemiological research and the next few years should witness rapid growth in knowledge and capacity to reduce the burden associated with these potentially serious mental disorders in young people.

References

Aggleton P, Hurry J, Warwick I (2000) *Young people and mental health.* Chichester, UK: Wiley.

American Psychiatric Association (1980) *DSM-III: Diagnostic and statistical manual of mental disorders* (3rd edn). Washington DC: American Psychiatric Association.

Andrews G (1999). Efficacy, effectiveness and efficiency in mental health service delivery. *Aust NZ J Psychiatry* 33:316–322.

Andrews G, Henderson S, eds (2000) *Unmet need in psychiatry. Problems, resources, responses.* Cambridge: Cambridge University Press.

Andrews G, Hall W, Teeson M, et al (1999) *The mental health of Australians.* Mental Health Branch, Commonwealth Department of Health and Age Care.

Bell RC, Dudgeon P, McGorry PD, et al (1998) The dimensionality of schizophrenia concepts in first episode psychosis. *Acta Psychiatr Scand* 97:334–342.

Biro V, Deane FP, Wilson C. (2002) *Illawarra and Shoalhaven survey of mental health care in general practice.* Wollongong, NSW: University of Wollongong, Illawarra Institute for Mental Health

Blashfield RK (1984) *The classification of psychopathology.* New York: Plenum.

Booth A, Crouter AC, Shanahan MJ (1999) *Transitions to adulthood in a changing economy. No work, no family, no future?* Westport, CT: Praeger.

Boyd JH, Burke JD, Gruenberg E, et al (1984) Exclusion criteria of DSM-111: A study of co-occurrence of hierarchy-free syndromes. *Arch Gen Psychiatry* 41:983–989.

Carlson GA, Fennig S, Bromet EJ (1994) The confusion between bipolar disorder and schizophrenia in youth: where does it stand in the 1990s? *J Am Acad Child Adolesc Psychiatry* 33:453–460.

Cuijpers P (2003) Examining the effects of prevention programs on the incidence of new cases of mental disorders: The lack of statistical power. *Am J Psychiatry,* 160:1385–1391.

Eaton WW (1995) Prodromes and precursors: epidemiologic data for primary prevention of disorders with slow onset. *Am J Psychiatry* 152:967–972.

Eaton WW (2001) *The sociology of mental disorders,* (3rd edn). Westport, CT: Praeger.

Fennig S, Kovasznay B, Rich C, et al (1994) Six-month stability of psychiatric diagnoses in first-admission patients with psychosis. *Am J Psychiatry* 151:1200–1208.

Ferdinand RF, van der Reijden M, Verhulst FC, et al (1995) Assessment of the prevalence of psychiatric disorder in young adults. *Br J Psychiatry* 166:480–488.

Frances A (1998) Problems in defining clinical significance in epidemiological studies. *Arch Gen Psychiatry* 55:119.

Goldberg D, Huxley P (1992) *Common mental disorders. A bio-social model.* London: Tavistock/Routledge.

Häfner H, Maurer W, Löffler B, et al (1995) Onset and early course of schizophrenia. In Häfner H, Gattaz WF, eds, *Search for the causes of schizophrenia.* New York: Springer: 43–66.

Jablensky A (1999) The 100-year epidemiology of schizophrenia. In Häfner H, Gattaz WF, eds, *Search for the causes of schizophrenia.* New York: Springer: 3–17.

Joyce PR (1984) Age of onset in bipolar affective disorder and misdiagnosis as schizophrenia. *Psychol Med* 14:145–149

Kessler RC, Foster CL, Saunders WB, et al (1995) Social consequences of psychiatric disorders: I. Educational attainment. *Am J Psychiatry* 152:1026–1031.

Keys Young (1997) *Research and consultation among young people on mental health issues: Final report.* Commonwealth Department of Health and Family Services, Canberra.

Kraemer HC, Yesavage JA, Taylor JL, et al (2000) How can we learn about developmental processes from cross-sectional studies, or can we? *Am J Psychiatry* 257:163–171.

Lincoln CV, McGorry PD (1999) Pathways to care in early psychosis: Clinical and consumer perspectives. In McGorry PD, Jackson HJ, eds, *The recognition and management of early psychosis: A preventive approach.* Cambridge University Press: 51–80.

McGorry PD (1991) Paradigm failure in functional psychosis: Review and implications. *Aust NZ J Psychiatry* 25:43–55.

McGorry P, Copolov DL, Singh BS (1989) The validity of the assessment of psychopathology in the psychoses. *Aust NZ J Psychiatry* 23:469–482.

McGorry P, Copolov DL, Singh BS (1990) Current concepts in functional psychosis: The case for a loosening of associations. *Schizophr Res* 3:221–234.

McGorry PD, Mihalopoulos C, Henry L, et al (1995) Spurious precision: Procedural validity of diagnostic assessment in psychotic disorders. *Am J Psychiatry* 152:220–223.

McGorry PD, Bell RC, Dudgeon PL, et al (1998) The dimensional structure of first episode psychosis: An exploratory factor analysis. *Psychol Med* 28:935–947.

McGorry PD, McKenzie D, Jackson HJ, et al (2000) Can we improve the diagnostic efficiency and predictive power of prodromal symptoms for schizophrenia? *Schizophr Res* 42:91–100

Mrazek PJ, Haggerty RJ (1994) *Reducing risks for mental disorders: Frontiers for preventive intervention research.* Washington DC: National Academy Press.

Murray C.J.L, Lopez AD (1996) *The global burden of disease: A comprehensive assessment of mortality and disability, injuries and risk factors in 1990 and projected to 2020.* Cambridge, MA: Harvard University Press.

Olfson M, Broadhead WE, Weissman MM, et al (1996) Subthreshold psychiatric symptoms in a primary care group practice. *Arch Gen Psychiatry* 53:880–886

Padmavathi R, Rajkumar S, Kumar N, et al (1998) Schizophrenic patients who were never treated: a study in an Indian urban community. *Psychol. Med* 28: 1113–1117.

Patton GC, Coffey C, Carlin JB, et al (2002) Cannabis use and mental health in young people: Cohort study. *BMJ* 325:1195–1198.

Regier DA, Kaelber CT, Rae DS, et al (1998) Limitations of diagnostic criteria and assessment instruments for mental disorders. *Arch Gen Psychiatry* 55:109–115.

Rose G (1992) *The strategy of preventive medicine.* Oxford University Press.

Rutter M (1998) Routes from research to clinical practice in child psychiatry: Retrospect and prospect. *J Child Psychol Psychiatry* 39:805–816.

Rutter M, Smith DJ, eds (1995) *Psychosocial disorders in young people: Time trends and their causes.* Chichester, UK: Wiley.

Ryle A (1995) *Cognitive analytic therapy: Developments in theory and practice.* Chichester, UK: Wiley.

Sawyer MG, Kosky RJ, Graetz BW, et al (2000) The National Survey of Mental Health and Wellbeing: the child and adolescent component. *Aust NZ J Psychiatry* 34:214–20

van Os J, Fahy TA, Jones P, et al (1996) Psychopathological syndromes in the functional psychoses: Associations with course and outcome. *Psychol Med* 26:161–76.

van Os J, Verdoux H, Bijl R, et al (1999a) Psychosis as an extreme of continuous variation in dimensions of psychopathology. In Gattaz WF, Häfner H, eds, *Search for the causes of schizophrenia, Vol. 4: Balance of the century.* New York: Springer: 59–80.

van Os JR, Ravelli A, Bijl RV (1999b) Evidence for a psychosis continuum in the general population. *Schizophr Res* 36:57.

van Os J, Hanssen M, Bijl RV, et al (2001) Prevalence of psychotic disorder and community level of psychotic symptoms. *Arch Gen Psychiatry* 58:663–668.

Verdoux H, Bergey C, Assens F, et al (1998) Prediction of duration of psychosis before first admission. *Eur Psychiatry* 13:346–352.

Warner R (2001) The prevention of schizophrenia: What interventions are safe and effective? *Schizophr Bull* **27**:551–562.

World Health Organization (1992) *International classification of disease: ICD-10* (10th edn). ICD-10. Ch V: Mental, behavioural and developmental disorders. Geneva: World Health Organization.

Wing JK, Cooper JE, Sartorius N (1974) *The measurement and classification of psychiatric symptoms.* Cambridge University Press.

Yung AR, McGorry PD (1996a) The prodromal phase of first-episode psychosis: Past and current conceptualizations. *Schizophr Bull* **22**:353–370.

Yung AR, McGorry PD (1996b) The initial prodrome in psychosis: Descriptive and qualitative aspects. *Aust NZ J Psychiatry* **30**:587–599.

Yung AR, Phillips LJ, Yuen HP, et al (2003) Psychosis prediction: 12 month follow-up of a high risk ('prodromal') group. *Schizophr Res* **60**:21–32

Zubrick SR, Silburn SR, Burton P, et al (2000) Mental health disorders in children and young people: Scope, cause and prevention. *Aust NZ J Psychiatry* **34**:570–578.

Appendix

COMPREHENSIVE ASSESSMENT OF AT RISK MENTAL STATES

(CAARMS)

POSITIVE SYMPTOM SCALES
and
ULTRA HIGH RISK
INTAKE CRITERIA

A. Yung, L. Phillips, P. McGorry, J. Ward, K. Donovan, K. Thompson

THE PACE CLINIC
University of Melbourne,
Department of Psychiatry
Melbourne, Australia

Patient Name:	CRF#:
Date:	Rater

Overview of the CAARMS

Aims:

- To determine if an individual meets the criteria for an 'At Risk Mental State'
- To rule out, or confirm criteria for acute psychosis
- To map a range of psychopathology and functioning factors, over time in young people at ultra high-risk of psychosis

Structure of the CAARMS:

- Ratings are made on a range of subscales that target different areas of psychopathology and functioning. From these ratings it is then possible to extract information relating to the above aims.

Overview of Symptoms and Functioning – Longitudinal Change:

- At the first interview (not follow-up interviews), the CAARMS aims to obtain a general overview of the history of change from the premorbid state in the respondent. All available information should be used.
- Record the **time of first noted change** – date and age of respondent in years:

  Date: …………….…………………………

  Age: ………………………..
- Note first ever symptoms or signs:

  …………………………………………..…….

  …………………………………………..…….

  ………………………………………………...

  ………………………………………………...
- Overview of course since then – map on timeline e.g.:

First change   Worst ever   Present state   Time

1: Positive Symptoms

1.1 Disorders Of Thought Content

Delusional Mood and Perplexity ('Non Crystallized Ideas')

- Have you had the feeling that something odd is going on that you can't explain? What is it like?
- Do you feel puzzled by anything? Do familiar surroundings feel strange?
- Do you feel that you have changed in some way?
- Do you feel that others, or the world, have changed in some way?

Non-Bizarre Ideas ('Crystallized Ideas')

- Ideas of Reference: Have you felt that things that were happening around you had a special meaning, or that people were trying to give you messages? What is it like? How did it start?
- Suspiciousness, Persecutory Ideas: Has anybody been giving you a hard time or trying to hurt you? Do you feel like people have been talking about you, laughing at you, or watching you? What is it like? How do you know this?
- Grandiose Ideas: Have you been feeling that you are especially important in some way, or that you have powers to do things that other people can't do?
- Somatic Ideas: Have you had the feeling that something odd is going on with your body that you can't explain? What is it like? Do you feel that your body has changed in some way, or that there is a problem with your body shape?
- Ideas of Guilt: Do you feel you deserve punishment for anything you have done wrong?
- Nihilistic Ideas: Have you ever felt that you, or a part of you, did not exist, or was dead? Do you ever feel that the world does not exist?
- Jealous Ideas: Are you a jealous person? Do you worry about relationships that your spouse/girlfriend/boyfriend has with other people?

- Religious Ideas: Are you very religious? Have you had any religious experiences?   _____
                                                                                                                          _____
- Erotomanic Ideas: Is anyone in love with you? Who?   _____
  How do you know this? Do you return his/her feelings?   _____

Bizarre Ideas ('Crystallized Ideas')

- Made thoughts, feelings, impulses: Have you felt that   _____
  someone, or something, outside yourself has been   _____
  controlling your thoughts, feelings, actions or urges?   _____
  Have you had feelings or impulses that don't seem to   _____
  come from yourself?   _____
- Somatic Passivity: Do you get any strange sensations in   _____
  your body? Do you know what causes them? Could it be   _____
  due to other people or forces outside yourself?   _____
- Thought Insertion: Have you felt that ideas or thoughts   _____
  that are not your own have been put into your head?   _____
  How do you know they are not your own? Where do   _____
  they come from?   _____
- Thought Withdrawal: Have you ever felt that ideas or   _____
  thoughts are being taken out of your head? How does   _____
  that happen?   _____
- Thought Broadcasting: Are your thoughts broadcast so   _____
  that other people know what you are thinking?   _____
- Thoughts Being Read: Can other people read your   _____
  mind?   _____

Disorders of Thought Content—Global Rating Scale

0 Never, absent	1 Questionable	2 Mild	3 Moderate	4 Moderately severe	5 Severe	6 Psychotic and severe
No disorders of thought content.	Mild elaboration of conventional beliefs as held by a proportion of the population	Vague sense that something is different, or not quite right with the world, a sense that things have changed but not able to be clearly articulated. Subject not concerned/ worried about this experience.	A feeling of perplexity. A stronger sense of uncertainty regarding thoughts than 2. **OR** Odd or unusual thoughts but whose content is not entirely implausible— may be some logical evidence. More evidence than rating of 4. Content of thoughts not original i.e. jealousy, mild paranoia.	Unusual thoughts, which can be easily dismissed. Clearly idiosyncratic beliefs, which although 'possible' have arisen without logical evidence. Less evidence than rating of 3 (eg referential ideas that certain events, objects or people have a particular and unusual significance.)	Unusual thoughts about which there is some doubt (not held with delusional conviction), or which the subject does not believe all the time. May result in some change in behaviour, but minor.	Unusual thoughts containing original and highly improbable material held with delusional conviction (no doubt). May have marked impact on behaviour.

Onset date:........................   Offset date:........................

Frequency and Duration

0	1	2	3	4	5	6
Absent	Less than once a month	Once a month to twice a week – **less** than one hour per occasion	Once a month to twice a week – **more** than one hour per occasion **OR** 3 to 6 times a week – **less** than one hour per occasion	3 to 6 times a week – **more** than an hour per occasion **OR** daily – **less** than an hour per occasion	Daily – **more** than an hour per occasion **OR** several times a day	Continuous

Pattern of Symptoms

0	1	2
No relation to substance use/stress noted	Occurs in relation to substance use/stress and at other times as well	Noted only in relation to substance use/stress

1.2 Perceptual Abnormalities

Visual Changes

- Distortions, illusions: Is there a change in the way things look to you? Do things somehow look different, or abnormal? Are there alterations in colour, or brightness of objects (things seeming brighter, or duller in colour)? Are there alterations in the size and shape of objects? Do things seem to be moving?
- Hallucinations: Do you have visions, or see things that may not really be there? Do you ever see things that others can't, or don't seem to? What do you see? At the time that you see these things, how real do they seem? Do you realise they are not real at the time, or only later?

_____
_____
_____
_____
_____
_____
_____
_____
_____
_____

Auditory Changes

- Distortions, illusions: Is there any change in the way things sound to you? Do things somehow sound different, or abnormal? Does your hearing seem more acute, or have increased sensitivity? Does your hearing seem muted, or less acute?
- Hallucinations: Do you ever hear things that may not really be there? Do you ever hear things that other people seem not to (such as sounds or voices)? What do you hear? At the time you hear these things, how real do they seem? Do you realise they are not real at the time, or only later?

_____
_____
_____
_____
_____
_____
_____
_____
_____
_____

Olfactory Changes

- Distortions, illusions: Does your sense of smell seem to be different, such as more, or less intense, than usual?
- Hallucinations: Do you ever smell things that other people don't notice? At the time, do these smells seem real? Do you realise they are not real at the time, or only later?

_____
_____
_____
_____
_____

Gustatory Changes

- Distortions, illusions: Does your sense of taste seem to be different, such as more, or less intense, than usual?
- Hallucinations: Do you ever get any odd tastes in your mouth? At the time that you taste these things, how real do they seem? Do you realise they are not real at the time, or only later?

_____

_____

_____

_____

_____

Tactile Changes

- Distortions, illusions, hallucinations: Do you ever get strange feelings on, or just beneath, your skin? At the time that you feel these things, how real do they seem? Do you realise they are not real at the time, or only later?

_____

_____

_____

_____

Somatic Changes

NOTE: Probes also used to rate Impaired Bodily Sensation, p.26

- Distortions, illusions: Do you ever get strange feelings in your body (eg feel that parts of your body have changed in some way, or that things are working differently)? Do you feel/think that there is a problem with some part, or all of your body, i.e. that it looks different to others, or is different in some way? How real does this seem?
- Hallucinations: Have you noticed any change in your bodily sensations, such as increased, or reduced intensity? Or unusual bodily sensations such as pulling feelings, aches, burning, numbness, vibrations?

_____

_____

_____

_____

_____

_____

_____

_____

_____

_____

Perceptual Abnormalities – Global Rating Scale

0 Never, absent	1 Questionable	2 Mild	3 Moderate	4 Moderately severe	5 Severe	6 Psychotic and severe
No abnormal perceptual experience.		Heightened, or dulled perceptions, distortions, illusions (eg lights/ shadows). Not particularly distressing. Hypnogogic/ hypnopompic experiences	More puzzling experiences: more intense/vivid distortions/ illusions, indistinct murmuring, fleeting shadows etc. Subject unsure of nature of experiences. Able to dismiss. Not distressing. Derealisation/ depersonali- sation	Much clearer experiences than 3 such as name being called, hearing phone ringing etc, but may be fleeting/ transient. Able to give plausible explanation for experience. May be associated with mild distress.	True hallucinations i.e. hearing voices or conversation, feeling something touching body. Subject able to question experience with effort. May be frightening or associated with some distress.	True hallucinations which the subject believes are true at the time of, and after, experiencing them. May be very distressing

Onset date:........................   *Offset date:*........................

Frequency and Duration

0	1	2	3	4	5	6
Absent	Less than once a month	Once a month to twice a week – **less** than one hour per occasion	Once a month to twice a week – **more** than one hour per occasion **OR** 3 to 6 times a week – **less** than one hour per occasion	3 to 6 times a week – **more** than an hour per occasion **OR** daily – **less** than an hour per occasion	Daily – **more** than an hour per occasion **OR** several times a day	Continuous

Pattern of Symptoms

0	1	2
No relation to substance use/stress noted	Occurs in relation to substance use/stress and at other times as well	Noted only in relation to substance use/stress

1.3 Disorganised Speech

NOTE: Probes also used to rate Alogia, p. 17

Subjective Change:

- Do you notice any difficulties with your speech, or ability to communicate with others?
- Do you have trouble finding the correct word at the appropriate time?
- Do you ever use words that are not quite right, or totally irrelevant?
- Have you found yourself going off on tangents when speaking and never getting to the point? Is this a recent change?
- Are you aware that you are talking about irrelevant things, or going off the track?
- Do other people ever seem to have difficulty in understanding what you are trying to say/trouble getting your message across?
- Do you ever find yourself repeating the words of others?
- Do you ever have to use gesture or mime to communicate due to trouble getting your message across? How bad is this?
- Does it ever make you want to stay silent and not say anything?

Objective Rating of Disorganised Speech

- Is it difficult to follow what the subject is saying at times due to using incorrect words, being circumstantial or tangential?
- Is the subject vague, overly abstract or concrete? Can responses be condensed?
- Do they go off the subject often and get lost in their words? Do they appear to have difficulty finding the right words?
- Do they repeat words that you have used or adopt strange words (or 'non-words') in the course of regular conversation?

Disorganised Speech— Global Rating Scale

0 Never, absent	1 Questionable	2 Mild	3 Moderate	4 Moderately severe	5 Severe	6 Psychotic and severe
Normal logical speech, no disorganisation, no problems communicating or being understood.		Slight subjective difficulties eg problems getting message across. Not noticeable by others.	Somewhat vague, some evidence of circumstantiality, or irrelevance in speech. Feeling of not being understood.	Clear evidence of mild disconnected speech and thought patterns. Links between ideas rather tangential. Increased feeling of frustration in conversation.	Marked circumstantiality, or tangentiality in speech, but responds to structuring in interview. May have to resort to gesture, or mime to communicate.	Lack of coherence, unintelligible speech, significant difficulty following line of thought. Loose associations in speech.

Onset date:.......................   *Offset date:.......................*

Frequency and Duration

0	1	2	3	4	5	6
Absent	Less than once a month	Once a month to twice a week – **less** than one hour per occasion	Once a month to twice a week – **more** than one hour per occasion OR 3 to 6 times a week – **less** than one hour per occasion	3 to 6 times a week – **more** than an hour per occasion OR daily – **less** than an hour per occasion	Daily – **more** than an hour per occasion OR several times a day	Continuous

Pattern of Symptoms

0	1	2
No relation to substance use/stress noted	Occurs in relation to substance use/stress and at other times as well	Noted only in relation to substance use/stress

8: Inclusion Criteria

Intake Criteria Checklist

<u>Group 1: Vulnerability Group</u> *This criterion identifies young people at risk of psychosis due to the combination of a trait risk factor and a significant deterioration in mental state and/or functioning*

	YES	NO
• **Family history of psychosis** in first degree relative <u>**OR**</u> **Schizotypal Personality Disorder** in identified patient	☐	☐
PLUS • **30% drop in GAF** score from premorbid level, sustained for a month	☐	☐
PLUS • **Change in functioning** occurred within last year and maintained at least a month	☐	☐
CRITERION MET FOR GROUP 1 – Vulnerability Group	☐	☐

<u>Group 2: Attenuated Psychosis Group</u> *This criterion identifies young people at risk of psychosis due to a subthreshold psychotic syndrome. That is, they have symptoms which do not reach threshold levels for psychosis due to subthreshold intensity (the symptoms are not severe enough) or they have psychotic symptoms but at a subthreshold frequency (the symptoms do not occur often enough).*

	YES	NO
2a) Subthreshold intensity:		
• **Severity Scale Score of 3–5** on *Disorders of Thought Content* subscale, **3–4** on *Perceptual Abnormalities* subscale **and/or 4–5** on *Disorganised Speech* subscales of the CAARMS	☐	☐
PLUS • **Frequency Scale Score of 3–6** on *Disorders of Thought Content, Perceptual Abnormalities* **and/or** *Disorganised Speech* subscales of the CAARMS for **at least a week** • <u>**OR**</u> **Frequency Scale Score of 2** on *Disorders of Thought Content, Perceptual Abnormalities* and *Disorganised Speech* subscales of the CAARMS **on more than two occasions**	☐	☐

	YES	NO
2b) Subthreshold frequency: • Severity Scale Score of 6 on *Disorders of Thought Content* subscale, 5–6 on *Perceptual Abnormalities* subscale and/or 6 on *Disorganised Speech* subscales of the CAARMS		
PLUS • Frequency Scale Score of 3 on *Disorders of Thought Content, Perceptual Abnormalities* **and/or** *Disorganised Speech* subscales of the CAARMS	☐	☐
PLUS (for both categories) • Symptoms present in past year and for not longer than five years	☐	☐
CRITERION MET FOR GROUP 2 – Attenuated Psychosis Group	☐	☐

<u>Group 3: BLIPS Group</u> *This criterion identifies young people at risk of psychosis due to a recent history of frank psychotic symptoms which resolved spontaneously (without antipsychotic medication) within one week.*

	YES	NO
• Severity Scale Score of 6 on *Disorders of Thought Content* subscale, **5 or 6** on *Perceptual Abnormalities* subscale **and/or** 6 on *Disorganised Speech* subscales of the CAARMS	☐	☐
PLUS • Frequency Scale Score of 4–6 on *Disorders of Thought Content, Perceptual Abnormalities* **and/or** *Disorganised Speech* subscales	☐	☐
PLUS • Each episode of symptoms is present for less than one week and symptoms spontaneously remit on every occasion.	☐	☐
PLUS • Symptoms occurred during last year and for not longer than five years	☐	☐
CRITERION MET FOR GROUP 3 – BLIPS Group	☐	☐

9: Psychosis Threshold /Anti-Psychotic Treatment Threshold

	YES	NO
• **Severity Scale Score of 6** on *Disorders of Thought Content* subscale, **5 or 6** on *Perceptual Abnormalities* subscale **and/or 6** on *Disorganised Speech* **subscales of the CAARMS**	☐	☐
PLUS		
• **Frequency Scale Score of greater than or equal to 4** on *Disorders of Thought Content, Perceptual Abnormalities* **and/or** *Disorganised Speech* subscales	☐	☐
PLUS		
• Symptoms present for **longer than one week**	☐	☐
PSYCHOSIS THRESHOLD CRITERION MET	☐	☐

Study Withdrawal ('Break Blind') Threshold

	YES	NO
• **Severity Scales Score of 5 or above** on *Aggression/Dangerous Behaviour* **and/or** *Suicidality/Self Harm* Subscales	☐	☐
• <u>NOTE:</u> This should be considered independently from level of psychosis		

Index

false positives, minimizing 25, 27–8, 29
  'multiple-gate' screening 28
  as retrospective concept 6, 12–13
  as risk factor for psychosis 25
  as symptomatic/detectable period 5–8
  symptoms, non-specific 7
  transition rates to psychosis 89, 90–1
  see also relapse prodrome
prospective studies 119
proton magnetic imaging of brains 98
psychoeducation 58–9
Psychological Assistance Service (PAS) 89
  transition rates to psychosis 91
psychological reaction to 'at risk' status 45
psychologists' roles in PACE Clinic 52
psychopathology
  in prospective recognition 27
  psychosis onset in UHR group 92–3
psychosis/psychotic disorder
  cortisol in 94
  criteria for UHR studies 91
  definition 19
  first episode
    duration of prodrome 23
    phases 6
  onset
    age and risk of onset 28
    associated factors in UHR group 92–6
    basic symptoms theory 23
    criteria 117
    defining 12, 15–20
    difficulty of recognizing symptoms 16
    as line of development 118
    neurobiology 94–102
    and pre-psychotic interventions 7, 8
    process of 19–20
  stress-vulnerability model 63
  as target syndrome 2
  transition rates from prodrome 89, 90–1
psychosis threshold in CAARMS 142

psychosocial decline 52
psychotherapy
  cognitive-behaviour oriented study 104
  cognitively oriented 63
  group 64
  plus risperidone 102–3
psychotic phase 6

quality of life 18–19

relapse
  and cannabis use 94
  case study 68–9
  and stress 96
relapse prodrome
  duration 23
  studies 20
research 82
  antipsychotics, use of 80
  clinical care
    distinguishing from 76, 82–3
    interaction with research 83
  clinical–research interface 75–86
  clinical trials 77–8
  confidentiality 76
  conflicts of interest 77
  consenting procedures 83–4
  costs/benefits 79–80
  designs 119
    future 122
  enriched samples 27
  findings 87–112
  focus of PACE Clinic 51
  guidelines
    draft, for UHR patients 70
    standard 76
  information
    provided to families 77, 79–80, 82, 84
    supplied to potential subjects 84
  introduction of staff 82